HOW TO HELP YOUR OVERWEIGHT CHILD...

eat healthily and well

enjoy exercise

boost self-esteem & self-respect

achieve a healthier weight

Karen Sullivan

RODALE

This edition first published in the UK in 2004 by
Rodale International Ltd
7–10 Chandos Street
London W1G 9AD
www.rodale.co.uk

© 2004 Karen Sullivan
All charts © Child Growth Foundation
Index compiled by Valerie Lewis Chandler

Printed and bound in the UK by CPI Bath using acid-free paper from sustainable sources.

1 3 5 7 9 8 6 4 2

A CIP record for this book is available from the British Library
ISBN 1-4050-7732-8

This paperback edition distributed to the book trade by Pan Macmillan Ltd

Notice
This book is intended as a reference volume only, not as a medical manual. The information given here is designed to help you make informed decisions about your child's health. It is not intended as a substitute for any treatment that they may have been prescribed by their doctor. If you suspect that they have a medical problem, we urge you to seek competent medical help.

Mention of specific companies, organizations or authorities in this book does not imply endorsement by the publisher, nor does mention of specific companies, organizations or authorities in the book imply that they endorse the book.

Addresses, websites and telephone numbers given in this book were accurate at the time the book went to press.

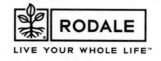

For Cole and Luke, who test-drove many
of my theories for practicality, and for Joe
and Ella, and the baby on the way!

Acknowledgements

A great many thanks are due to the huge number of people who have commented upon and helped me with this book. I have been struck by the unbelievable commitment that so many health professionals have to understanding the many causes of childhood obesity and coming up with realistic and practical guidelines for doctors, parents and organizations to adopt.

First and foremost, I would like to thank Tam Fry, Honorary Chairman of the Child Growth Foundation in the UK. His commitment to this project has been unprecedented, and I owe him many thanks.

Thanks too to Dr Ian Campbell, President of the National Obesity Forum, a nationwide network of doctors and nurses promoting 'best practice' in the management of overweight. He has shown support and enthusiasm from the outset, and been an enormous help in all areas.

Dr Tim Lobstein of the International Obesity Task Force, and Director of the Food Commission in the UK, advised on some key areas that affect childhood obesity and highlighted the role that parents can play in fighting the scourge of advertising aimed at children. Thank you, Tim.

Dr Tim Cole, of the Institute of Child Health, has also been extremely helpful, and has put me in touch with key experts in the area of childhood obesity. Thanks are also due to Dr Susan Jebb, head of Nutrition & Health Research at MRC Human Nutrition Research, and expert on so many facets of childhood overweight and obesity, and to Dr Michael Apple.

Many organizations have also given support and assistance, including the British Nutrition Foundation, the British Dietetic Association, the Association for the Study of Obesity (ASO), the International Obesity Task Force, the Food and Drink Federation, the World Health Organization, the Eating Disorders Association (EDA) and the Royal College of Paediatrics and Child Health, among many others. Thanks, too, to the many children who shared their stories, and how they felt about having a weight problem.

Special thanks are due to my editor at Rodale, Anne Lawrance, who has shown considerable patience, enthusiasm and insight throughout this project; to Jillian Stewart for excellent editing and input, as well as an amazing ability to remain unflappable in the light of unexpected last-minute changes; to Davina Russell for organizing the website www.youroverweightchild.org; and finally to Margot Weale at Midas, for her efforts in getting this book out to all the right people.

Finally, thank you to my partner Max, who has been supportive and encouraging as I wrote this book while heavily pregnant, and to my children, Luke and Cole, who were interested and enthusiastic throughout, despite the long hours I spent at my computer.

Contents

Foreword

Few people can have failed to notice that we are in the midst of a rapid growth in childhood obesity, with all the added problems that can bring. The press is full of endless stories, statistics and government reports labelling us as a nation of over-eating and lazy families and forecasting huge costs both to the individual sufferer and to our health services. But is it really that bad? Are we really living in an age when children will start to be outlived by their parents? That we are in the midst of a major challenge to the health of our children is not in doubt. Being overweight now affects one in three children in the United Kingdom and obesity, or serious overweight, has reached epidemic levels. Among pre-school children as many as nine per cent are now obese, and by the age of 15 years, that level has risen to 17 per cent, or one in eight teenagers. By the time we reach adulthood as many as one in five of us is clinically obese. The consequences are alarming. Already, the majority of those obese children will have an increased risk of disease, with early risk markers for heart disease and diabetes, high blood pressure and raised cholesterol being present in two-thirds. And of course we must not overlook the social or psychological impact of being overweight on a child who is teased or bullied at school.

Being aware of the problem is one thing. But what can a concerned parent do to reduce the risk of his or her child becoming overweight, or indeed help them achieve a healthier weight if a problem already exists? Where can a worried mum or dad turn for advice and support for their child? And ultimately, whose responsibility is it to tackle the problem? In reality, it must be everyone's responsibility. Not just parents, but the education system, food manufacturers, retailers and advertisers, the media, the medical professions, and local and national government. The view from Government is that their role is not to enforce health on children, rather to empower children – and their parents – to take control and responsibility for their own health. Government is taking action, but for children affected by overweight now any measures taken by government or industry may not happen quickly enough. Our health services are not able to deliver the support and advice parents and their children need. Schools are trying very hard to cope with all the academic demands placed upon them, let alone focus on health, though they are more involved in delivering health education now than ever before and can be an immensely influential force for good. The reality is that health must start at home. Parents need to be the foundation stone on which their child's health and well-being is built. And the most crucial, the most basic element of that well-being must be a healthy lifestyle, with good nutrition and plenty of enjoyable exercise.

How to Help Your Overweight Child will be a welcome addition to any parent's bookshelf. It intelligently explores not just the obvious causes of overweight in children – that is, eating more than is needed and not being active enough – but looks in detail at the potential underlying reasons in a child's life that make weight gain more likely, reasons often beyond the child's immediate control. Reading this book will help parents make a calm but detailed assessment of their child's risk of overweight, and their risk of developing some of the medical problems we know can develop as a result of their overweight. But this book does much more than simply raise awareness of the problem. It actually tells the concerned parent what they can do, where to start, and where to get extra help if needed. Karen Sullivan provides a host of sensible, practical, well researched and child-friendly suggestions to allow parents to help their child regain control over their health, to eat healthily but still have fun, to become more active and to enjoy life more. Staying at a healthy weight isn't easy. In fact it's extremely difficult, but this book promises to be an invaluable aid to anyone who wants to work with their child to maximize their health both now, and into the future.

Dr Ian W Campbell
President of the National Obesity Forum

Introduction

It's not easy to admit that your child has a weight problem and, not surprisingly, many parents choose to keep the matter private, or to overlook it altogether. After all, as nurturers and primary carers, having an overweight child seems to be a poor reflection on our parenting skills and our ability to control our children's diets and lifestyle habits. Moreover, with the intense media focus on slimming and achieving the 'perfect' body, weight problems are, well, rather *embarrassing*.

Recently, however, the top has been blown off that particular can of worms, for not only are a huge percentage of children now considered overweight, even obese, but the scale of the problem is reaching epidemic proportions. The World Health Organization has called it the 'biggest unrecognized health problem in the world'. And not even the most damning critics can blame a problem of that magnitude on poor parenting.

The bottom line is: if you have an overweight child, you are not alone, and certainly not solely to blame. There are various factors that can lead to a child becoming overweight or obese and many of them are a unique product of life in our modern age. However, regardless of the cause – and I will, of course, look at the causes in detail – we, as parents, have a responsibility to do something about our overweight children.

So what's going on? Is overweight in childhood really that serious a problem?

Many of us struggle with our own weight, attempting to keep it within some sort of limit through various means. At some point in our lives, most of us will have tried fad diets without much long-term success and toyed with becoming regular visitors to the gym or swimming pool, but it's usually a battle that fails to reap many rewards – and it's certainly not a war that we'd want to foist on our children. It's hard, too, to imagine why it would be necessary. Chubby-cheeked babies are infinitely more attractive than those who are thin, and cherubic children with dimpled knees are positively delightful. But when does 'plump' become unattractive, and at what stage are children expected to transform from sweet little dumplings into slim tots?

Let's get one thing straight, right from the outset – the average child is not perfectly slim. Throughout various stages of development, puppy fat accumulates and then is dispersed. Some children are big-boned, with an uneven weight distribution; others are skinny and every extra pound gained looks out of place on them. Even the most beautiful baby will go through unattractive periods, and the most wiry child will lay down a few extra pounds in advance of a growth spurt. Like adults, children come in all shapes and sizes and there is no 'norm' or Holy Grail to which you should aspire. Be aware, too, that although images of skinny models grace almost every magazine cover, being underweight is not healthy either and can cause problems for children that are every bit as serious as overweight.

When I talk about overweight I'm not referring to a few extra pounds but excess weight that can damage health. Later in this book we'll look at how to assess whether your child really is overweight, or just laying down fat in the natural course of growing up. So don't assume the worst if your once sprightly child has developed a bit of a tummy or chubby cheeks. But equally, don't bury your head in the sand. If you've bought this book, chances are you are concerned about your child's weight, and parental instinct is a pretty strong divining rod when it comes to assessing potential problems with our children. If you think there is a problem, there may well be one – and you are wise to be concerned.

The scale of the problem

According to the International Obesity Task Force, some 22 million of the world's under-fives are overweight or obese. And you may be surprised to learn that the problem isn't confined to Western countries. In Zambia and Morocco, for example, between 15 and 20 per cent of four-year-olds are obese. And in Chile, Peru and Mexico, obesity rates are running at more than 25 per cent among children aged between four and 10.

In the UK, the government estimates that the number of overweight children has increased by 25 per cent since 1995, with an average of almost 17 per cent of UK children now classified as obese. Obesity among six-year-olds has doubled in recent years to 8.5 per cent and trebled to around 17 per cent among 15-year-olds – and note, these figures are for 'obese' children; not those who are simply overweight. Some leading medical experts warn that in excess of one in three adults, one in five boys and one in three girls will be obese by 2020 if current trends continue.

In Australia the figures are better for obesity but they're little different when it comes to overweight: about 23 per cent of Australian children and adolescents are affected by overweight and obesity, with six per cent being obese. However, researchers point out that these are conservative estimates, as there has been no systematic monitoring of the prevalence of overweight and obesity in Australian children and adolescents since 1995. Significantly, over the previous decade, the number of overweight children almost doubled and the number of obese children more than tripled.

In New Zealand a national study, published in 2003, found almost one in three children aged five to 14 were overweight or obese. And a quarter of South African children between the ages of 12 and 18 are now classified as being overweight or obese, and this despite the fact that malnutrition is still rife in the country. In the US, 25 per cent of white children (of all ages) are overweight, and that figure rises to 33 per cent in the African American and Hispanic populations.

These frightening statistics illustrate just how many nations are teetering on the brink of an obesity epidemic – indeed it could be said that we're already in the thick of it. But while it can be comforting for parents to learn that they are not alone, there is no doubt that this is a wake-up call for us all. Obesity is not just a condition that defines the way a child looks, it's a serious threat to their health – and here's why.

The health implications

Obesity is implicated in many, many health conditions. Much of the research has been undertaken in adults, as obesity and overweight in children is still a relatively recent phenomenon. But the facts remain the same: any overweight person, regardless of their age, is at risk of health problems, and some of them are very serious indeed.

Cancer

A 2003 study found that the more overweight a person is, the higher their chance of developing many types of cancer. The American Cancer Society study, which tracked 900,000 people over 16 years, found excess weight to be a likely factor in 20 per cent of all cancer deaths in women and 14 per cent in men.

A range of cancers, including stomach, prostate and cervix cancers, have been found to have some link to weight. Fat raises the amount of oestrogen in the blood, increasing the risk of cancers in the female reproductive system (that includes cancers of the breast, ovaries, cervix and uterus) and it increases the risk of acid reflux, which is linked to cancer of the oesophagus. The same study also found that obesity is directly linked to non-Hodgkin's lymphoma, cancers of the pancreas and liver and, in men, the stomach and prostate.

With children becoming overweight at increasingly younger ages, this could mean susceptibility to serious forms of cancer that normally appear in later life – and a much shorter lifespan.

Diabetes

Type 2 diabetes is a condition normally associated with obese and overweight adults – hence it is often referred to as 'adult-onset' diabetes. However, some 45 per cent of newly diagnosed cases of childhood diabetes are type 2. And of children diagnosed with type 2 diabetes, 85 per cent are obese. A new study suggests that one in four overweight children is already showing early signs of type 2 diabetes. In fact, the World Health Organization has made the grim prediction that if the global obesity epidemic continues, 300 million people could have type 2 diabetes by the year 2024.

Type 2 diabetes is a lifelong (chronic) disease in which the pancreas cannot produce enough insulin and/or the body tissues become resistant to insulin. Basically, insulin is necessary for the body to utilize and store energy. It does this by controlling the level of sugar in the blood. When the mechanism fails because not enough insulin is available or it is not being properly utilized, the blood sugar level must be controlled through diet. Children who are overweight, are not physically active and have a close relative with type 2 diabetes are most at risk of the disease. Most children with type 2 diabetes do not have symptoms when the disease is diagnosed – it is usually discovered when the child sees a health professional for another reason. If symptoms are present, they are usually mild – an increase in frequency of urination, a rise in levels of thirst and a slight weight loss. So you may not be aware of the problem until your child visits the doctor for another reason. Many cases of type 2 diabetes are diagnosed during adolescence, however experts are now seeing cases of diabetes in children as young as four.

Diabetes doesn't go away. If your child acquires the disease, it is his for life – and your child will be on a special diet for life. If the disease is not controlled, it can damage the eyes, heart, kidneys, blood vessels and nerves. A long-term study of 51 Canadian patients aged 18 to 33, who had been diagnosed with type 2 diabetes before the age of 17, found that seven had died of diabetes-related illnesses, three others were on dialysis, one had become blind at the age of 26 and one had had a toe amputation. Of 56 pregnancies over the course of the study, only 35 had resulted in live births.

Heart disease

Heart disease has many causes, but there is little doubt that being overweight makes a child more susceptible to it. A ground-breaking study of overweight children found that the majority of those studied had at least one additional risk factor for developing heart disease, such as high cholesterol levels or high blood pressure, and 20 per cent had two or more additional risk factors.

Recent evidence has also found that the arteries of overweight children can be in as poor condition as those of middle-aged smokers. This could make them up to five times more likely than those of normal weight to have a heart attack or stroke before age 65. There is also evidence that some overweight children already have a build-up of fatty deposits in key arteries and that some smaller arteries may be blocked. In other words, many children are on target for a heart attack already. According to Dr George Blackburn, associate director of the Division of Nutrition at Harvard Medical School, 'We must intensify efforts for early identification and early prevention of overweight and obesity, or we are going to have the first generation of children who are not going to live as long as their parents'.

To make matters worse, it appears that metabolic syndrome – a constellation of conditions that together raise the risk of heart disease – affects far more children than previously thought. Also known as syndrome X, the condition is generally diagnosed when the following conditions are present: insulin resistance, abdominal obesity based on waist circumference (or, in children, a high body mass index), high blood pressure, low 'good' cholesterol and high triglycerides (blood fats). The underlying causes for metabolic syndrome are being overweight or obese, being physically inactive and having a genetic predisposition. A study carried out in 2004 found that the prevalence of metabolic syndrome increased as kids got heavier. Overall, 38.7 per cent of moderately obese participants and 49.7 per cent of severely obese participants had metabolic syndrome. However, none of the overweight or non-obese children and adolescents who took part had the syndrome.

Studies of the relationship between heart disease and weight show that excess weight can cause serious heart problems that reduce quality of life and lead to an early death. And while most studies have involved overweight adults, with more and more children now suffering the same risk factors as overweight adults, we could be looking at heart attacks and strokes occurring in very young adults.

High blood pressure

This is one of the side-effects of overweight, and one of the risk factors for heart disease. As your child puts on weight, he gains mostly fatty tissue. Just like other parts of the body, this tissue relies on oxygen and nutrients in the blood to survive. Hence as demand for oxygen and nutrients increases, the amount of blood circulating through the arteries also increases. And more blood travelling through the arteries means added pressure on the artery walls. Weight gain also typically causes an increase in the level of insulin, the blood-sugar-controlling hormone in the blood, and an increase in insulin is associated with retention of sodium (salt) and water, which again increases blood volume. In addition, excess weight is often associated with an increase in heart rate and a reduction in the capacity of the blood vessels to transport blood. All of these factors can cause an increase in blood pressure.

Is this really a problem? A study released in 2004 found that blood pressure levels for children and teenagers have risen substantially since 1988. And according to an earlier study, for each 1- to 2-millimetre rise in their systolic blood pressure, children face a 10 per cent greater risk of developing hypertension as a young adult. This leaves them more likely to suffer heart disease and strokes, at increasingly younger ages. Although it's normally very uncommon in children, raised blood pressure occurs nine times more frequently in obese children and teenagers than in those who are not obese. However, it's worth noting that changes made when a child is young can completely reverse the damage, which gives parents every reason to address weight issues now.

Osteoarthritis

This joint disorder most often affects the knees, hips and lower back. Excess weight puts extra pressure on these joints and wears away the cartilage that protects them, resulting in joint pain and stiffness. It's a serious condition, and profoundly affects quality of life. Children who are overweight are at increased risk of developing osteoarthritis at a younger age. They are also at greater risk of developing back pain, one of the commonest health problems caused or exacerbated by overweight and obesity.

Sleep apnoea

This too is a serious problem, and one that is on the increase – particularly among those who are obese.

Sleep apnoea occurs when a person stops breathing for short periods – around 10 seconds or more – while asleep. Because of increased weight, and fat around the neck area, the soft tissue in the throat intermittently blocks the airways during sleep. These breathing stoppages can occur up to a hundred times a night, leading to memory problems, headaches and fatigue, all of which obviously have a knock-on effect on a child's ability to concentrate at school. Some experts consider the condition to be literally 'choking on fat'.

Night-time symptoms include snoring, breathing pauses during sleep, restless sleep and mouth breathing. In the daytime, you may notice your child has difficulty getting up in the morning, even after getting the normal amount of sleep, is hyperactive, inattentive, and exhibits behaviour problems and sleepiness.

You may think that a sleep disorder can't be dangerous, but it is – it has been linked to high blood pressure and to increased chances of heart disease, stroke and irregular heart rhythms (arrhythmias). Unfortunately, not all of the long-term effects of untreated sleep apnoea are known, but specialists generally agree that the effects are harmful. If nothing else, the continual lack of quality sleep can affect your child's life in many ways, including causing depression, irritability, loss of memory and a lack of energy.

Self-esteem problems

The most immediate consequences of being overweight during child-hood and adolescence are psychosocial. Obese and overweight children have low self-esteem and body dissatisfaction. They are also more likely to underachieve academically, have poor job prospects and be socially isolated. Research shows that obese children feel that being overweight is a worse disability than losing a limb.

The economic time bomb

It may seem a rather cold way of looking at it, but it is important to be aware that chronic health conditions take an enormous toll on our health services, and that has to be paid for out of taxpayers' pock-ets. If current trends continue, our children will be forced to fund the serious health consequences of an increasingly overweight pop-ulation. And if there is a shortfall, there simply won't be money in the pot for research and treatment of other health conditions. So if your child becomes ill as an adult, there may not be enough money to pay for his care.

Recent estimates suggest that between two and eight per cent of the total sick-care costs in Western countries are attributable to obesity. The direct cost of treating obesity in England in 2002 is esti-mated to be £46–49 million, while the costs of treating the conse-quences of obesity are an estimated £945–1,075 million. That's a lot of money and much of it could be spent on researching diseases for which there is currently no cure.

Is it all bad news?

The fact is that overweight adolescents have a 70 per cent chance of becoming overweight or obese adults, so if you don't do something to halt your child's weight gain, their quality of life will be seriously affected. Overweight is a serious issue and it's vital not to play down the potential consequences. One recent study has concluded that 'Mortality attributable to excess weight is a major public health problem in the EU. At least one in 13 annual deaths in the EU is likely to be related to excess weight.' In the EU, the UK has the highest individual percentage of all, with 8.7 per cent of deaths being attributable to excess weight.

However, studies do show that changing eating habits, adopting a healthier lifestyle, including increasing exercise and reducing sedentary activities, can make a dramatic difference – and even reverse the damage caused by overweight. Take one of the studies I outlined earlier, in which the arteries of overweight children were found to be similar to those of a 45-year-old who has been smoking for at least 10 years. Researchers also found that changing to a healthy diet and adding daily exercise not only meant that the overweight children studied lost weight, but their arteries also became healthier. Researcher, Professor Kam Woo said 'We were surprised that the children had developed vascular abnormalities at such a young age, and by how readily these could be reversed with simple lifestyle measures.'

So the message is that it's never too late. Even very obese children can learn to eat properly and change their lifestyles to promote good health. And this book will show you how to do just that.

Many parents are genuinely bewildered by weight problems in children who have previously been healthy and well, and surprised to find that children who eat much the same as their friends suddenly and inexplicably pile on pounds.

So, how do you encourage a child to change lifelong habits, particularly when they form part of our popular culture? How can a faddy eater be persuaded to eat fruit and vegetables and forgo his favourite chips and crisps? How can you shift kids away from the TV or games console and out into the park, on to bikes, or involve them in sports when they've developed sedentary habits? Most importantly, perhaps, how do you deal with the feelings your child might be experiencing if she has become overweight? Her self-esteem may be low; she may have a poor body image and be embarrassed about her size; and she may not want to draw attention to herself or her body by taking part in activities where she may lose face.

It's worth considering too whether your child genuinely is overweight, or if he's just experiencing weight gain as a precursor to growth – or if your child's weight gain is due to factors outside normal parameters.

Whatever the cause, this book will help you identify if your child has a weight problem, assess the causes that are unique to your child, and show you how to work together *as a family* to right them before ill-health – on both a physical and emotional level – sets in. We'll look at practical ways to make changes so that your child both looks well and feels good about himself. It's not always easy on a tight budget and an even tighter daily schedule to make the necessary adjustments, but there are ways round it and we'll look at how to work together to manage the family timetable and change the dynamic to one that is more positive and conducive to healthy family living. And it is vital that the whole family gets involved – otherwise, quite frankly, it won't work.

If you come up against problems, there's a chapter devoted to troubleshooting – how to deal with relapses, comfort eating, peer pressure, embarrassment and more. You'll find advice on getting support and back-up for when the going gets tough and there's also an invaluable list of organizations that can help you and your child.

Unlike many health problems, obesity and overweight can be successfully addressed by making some changes to the way you and your family live. There are no quick-fix solutions, but the adjustments you make can transform your lives, and enhance well-being on all levels. Every parent wants a happy, healthy future for their children, but obesity poses an unprecedented threat to that future. The sooner you work out the problems and make the necessary adjustments, the better. And that process starts now.

Chapter One

Is Your Child Overweight?

Most parents are conscious of weight gain in their children, and fairly switched on when it comes to assessing a potential problem. Throughout childhood, weight can fluctuate dramatically, all within normal bounds. Weight increases in advance of puberty, for example, and during other periods of growth. In the winter months some children put on a little weight, which naturally disperses when they are more active during the summer. Periods of stress or emotional problems, illness or injuries, can also affect eating habits and activity levels, causing weight gain. These too may be short-term situations that affect a child's weight, and are resolved when the causative factors are addressed.

While it is undoubtedly important to keep tabs on even small gains in weight, it is also important to keep things in perspective and not to panic or worry unduly. If you keep an eye on your child's diet and exercise levels, as well as any factors that might be affecting his or her emotional health, small problems will not become big ones.

There is no doubt, though, that weight gain can be insidious and can creep up without you having noticed. Some parents state that they first noticed that their child had put on too much weight when they saw them in a swimming costume, next to other, slimmer children, or they suddenly realized that toddler puppy fat had expanded into something quite different. It doesn't make you a bad parent to have missed the signs – in fact, many of us fail to notice weight gain in ourselves until our clothes become too tight. And if you've missed an unhealthy gain in weight, or don't have a realistic picture of your child's overall weight, you are not alone. A ground-breaking study released in the UK in 2004, found that even when their children are clinically obese, at least one-third of parents – particularly fathers – believe they are the normal weight for their age. It's not easy to dispassionately judge someone we love, particularly when we see them every day and become accustomed to their appearance – but there's also some truth to the idea that we close our eyes to the things we don't want to see.

However, it's never too late to open your eyes and make an honest assessment. The key is to work out whether your child is genuinely overweight – using the methods outlined on the following pages – and then take steps to address the lifestyle factors that might be contributing to that weight gain.

In this chapter we'll look at the various ways of assessing a child's weight. We'll also examine how you can pinpoint whether or not weight could potentially be an issue in future, by assessing overall eating habits and lifestyle factors. It's certainly a lot easier to prevent a problem in children than it is to try and rectify one. Weight is an emotive issue and one that has dramatic effects on self-esteem and self-image, which are crucial to a child's emotional development. The earlier you address the problem, and the more sensitively you do so, the more successful you are likely to be.

There are many ways to work out whether or not your child is overweight, and some are more reliable than others. The important thing is not to draw unnecessary attention to what you may perceive to be a problem. Your child will be as aware as you are of any potential weight problem, and dealing with it in a clinical manner will only undermine their self-confidence. Many families regularly measure their children's height, and measuring weight as part of the proceedings is an easy way to keep an eye on potential weight problems without making it an issue. You will then have the data you need to make an assessment privately, and come up with an action plan that doesn't make your child feel under scrutiny, or 'different'. Obviously children must be involved in any programme to adjust their weight, and that's something we'll look at later in this book, but their role must be considered carefully and sensitively.

What is overweight?

This may sound like a silly question, but many parents are quite understandably confused by the terminology. Obesity and overweight are two terms used frequently in the media, and it can be difficult to discern the difference between them, or the importance of either. Various studies have been undertaken to determine what exactly constitutes overweight and obesity in both children and adults. Children in particular have been hard to categorize, mainly because of the vast differences in the way that they grow and the timing of that growth.

Strictly speaking, overweight is simply an excess of weight for a child's height. However, various factors can affect weight, including having a larger, heavier bone structure and more muscle, and these factors are not taken into account when overweight is assessed in this way. Therefore, your child's weight may be way off the growth charts for his height, but he may look slim and healthy. In this case, use a little common sense. A heavy child is not necessarily a fat child, even if he weighs more than average for his height.

In essence then overweight is really only a problem when there is an excess of body fat. A child who is overweight and carrying too much fat could be on the route to obesity – and that's where health problems really begin.

What is obesity?

Strictly speaking, obesity is defined as an excess of body fat. Excess body fat adds additional weight to a child and can cause a deviation from normal growth. If your child is gaining weight more rapidly than normal, he should be checked for obesity.

The height and build of the child affects whether he or she is considered obese at a given weight. A child usually is obese when he is significantly over the ideal body weight for his height. In general, if a child's weight is 20 per cent or more in excess of the expected weight for a given height, they may be obese. Most parents will have growth charts in the record books supplied by their doctor or health visitor when their child was born, or in the back of childcare books. (Unfortunately, the latest charts are too large and complex to enable them all to be reproduced in any usable form here.)

Growth charts

Growth charts give you an indication of where your child falls on the scale in relation to his peers. They are one way of keeping tabs on height and weight, but more than that they are an important tool for monitoring children's development. The percentile curves on these charts represent the percentage of children who are the same height or weight. The 50th percentile represents the median, or average, height or weight for each age group – hence 50 per cent of children will be above this point and 50 per cent will be below it. If a 3½-year-old boy, for example, weighed around 13.5 kg, then he would be at the 9th percentile for his weight at this age (the sample chart opposite illustrates how his centile band is arrived at). This means that 91 per cent of boys his age weigh more than him, but it also means that he weighs more than eight per cent of boys of this same age.

How your child has been growing is more important than what percentile he is in. Children at or below the 9th percentile for weight may be normal if their growth velocity, or the rate at which they are growing, is normal. Children that are small with a normal growth pattern will have their own growth curve on the growth chart but it will still be parallel to the 9th percentile. It is important to look at a number of different values of height and weight over time to assess a child's rate of development.

In terms of keeping tabs on weight, what you are looking for is a consistent curve. If your child suddenly jumps from the 50th to the 91st percentile in weight, there may be a problem. In contrast, if your child has always been in the 91st percentile on the charts, continues to be, and shows no sign of excess weight, there is no need for concern.

You may already have a set of growth charts on which you have charted your child's growth. While it can be normal for children to change percentiles between birth and 18 months of age, after this age they usually follow their growth curves fairly closely (within one or two centile bands). Any big shift can represent an unhealthy change in weight.

If you haven't kept a record of your child's height and weight across the years, it's not too late to start, and it's a good way to

Weight-for-age and Height-for-age percentiles
Boys aged 1–5 years

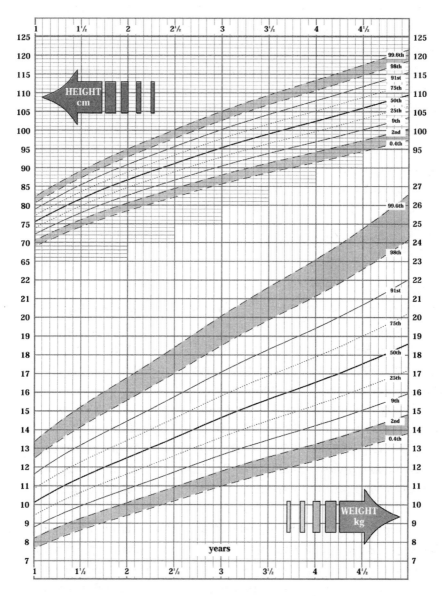

monitor both growth and potential problems. If you find your child is already well above the 91st percentile in weight for their height, and you are concerned that they seem overweight, now is the time to take action.

BMI charts

BMI – body mass index, a measurement derived from someone's weight and height – was only recently recommended as an additional routine measurement of growth.

From the age of one you can plot your child's BMI on a standard chart, which shows those of other children the same age. Because what is normal changes with age (young children have more 'baby fat', for instance), children's BMI measurements must be plotted on paediatric BMI charts rather than assessed using the universal normal range for BMI, as is done with adults.

Sounds complicated? It's not. If you've ever done your own adult calculation, you'll know that there are standard figures which tell you whether you are underweight, normal, overweight or obese. In adults, a BMI of under 18.5 is considered to be underweight, 18.5–24.9 to be healthy, 25–29.9 to be overweight and 30 or over to be obese.

However, because of the way children grow it's impossible to categorize them so easily, although you use the same equation – weight in kilograms divided by height in metres squared. For example, a seven-year-old boy who weighs 25 kg and is 1.1 m tall has a BMI of 20.6 (1.1 x 1.1 = 1.21; 25 ÷ 1.21 = 20.6) but is definitely overweight. Also, as you will also see from the chart opposite, BMI declines from infancy to about five or six years of age, and then increases with age through childhood and adolescence. Kids tend to stick fairly closely to the same line throughout their childhood, and you will want to establish that this is the case with your child.

After the age of five or six, the rise in BMI is called 'adiposity rebound' and this is a period that doctors watch quite carefully. If adiposity rebound occurs too early (at around the age of three or four, for example), studies show that a child may have a higher risk of overweight in late adolescence and early adulthood. If the adiposity rebound occurs too late, your doctor may be concerned as to whether your child is putting on enough weight. If the rebound is too steep – weight is put on too quickly for your child's height – it's time to take a look at what your child is eating, and his activity levels, to ascertain if either of these are at the root of the increase in weight.

Boys BMI chart
Birth to 20 years

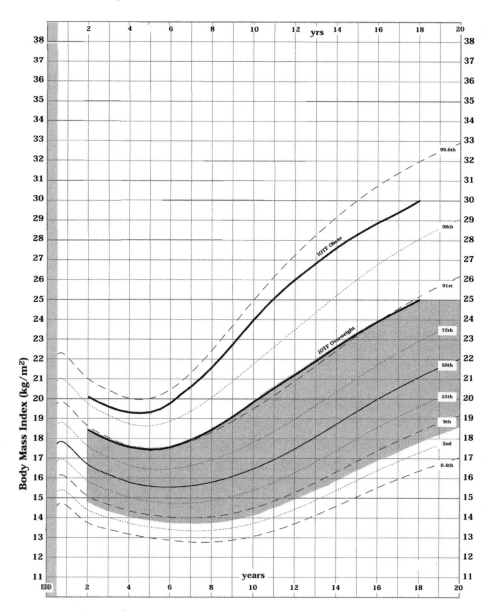

What do these charts mean?

The BMI charts for boys and girls show the standard centile lines for
BMI derived from UK data. The grey shaded area indicates a healthy

Girls BMI chart
Birth to 20 years

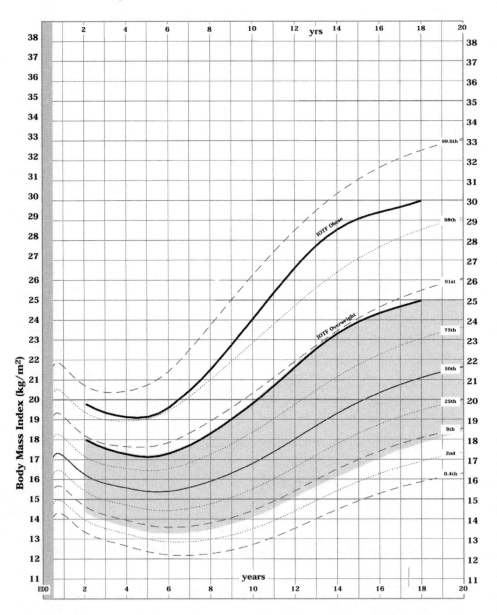

BMI range. The International Obesity Task Force (IOTF) lines equate with WHO adult definitions of obesity and overweight in adults.

When you try to decipher BMI readings, it's important to look at them as a trend instead of focusing on individual numbers. Any one measurement, taken out of context, might give you the wrong impression of your child's growth. The real value of BMI measurements lies in viewing them as a pattern over time. Your child may be growing normally and be well within a healthy weight even if her weight climbs to a higher growth curve – as long as the curve doesn't keep on climbing. For example, if she shifts from the 50th to the 75th percentile but remains there, she is probably growing in a way that is right for her.

Keep your eye on the curve as your child gets older and watch for blips. Again, if you haven't kept a record of your child's weight and height across the years, you can start now.

BMI charts are carefully designed to take into account normal weight gain during periods of growth. However, BMI is not a direct or perfect measure of body fat. A very muscular child, for example, may find themselves in the overweight category – because muscle weighs a lot more than fat. For this reason, experts now recommend that a child's waist measurement is taken to give a more accurate picture. A high waist centile in conjunction with a high BMI centile will confirm fatness more conclusively. You will find the waist circumference charts on pages 10–11. The shaded area represents a healthy waist range.

Note, there are separate BMI and waist measurement charts for boys and girls to account for differences in growth rates and amounts of body fat as the two genders mature. So make sure you check your child's BMI – and, if necessary, waist circumference – on the right chart!

A less scientific approach

A child's appearance should offer some pretty good clues as to whether or not they are overweight, and a quick investigation into their eating habits and activity levels is probably all the evidence you need to confirm suspicions.

Beyond the age of two, no child should have rolls of fat anywhere on their body and certainly not on their midriff. If you can see and count their ribs, there is no cause for alarm. Musculature should be evident in most healthy children (that is, you should be able to see muscles beneath the skin, small as they might be), as should some evidence of a skeleton! From the age of about six, weight

Boys waist circumference

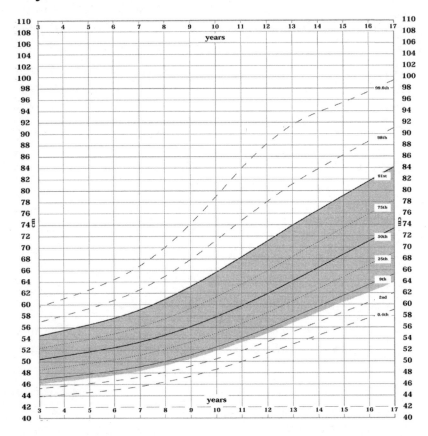

begins to fall from the arms and legs (the extremities) and settle around the trunk. So if your seven-year-old is carrying too much weight around his thighs or upper arms, chances are he is overweight. In a moment we'll look at normal weight gain in children, and where the fat stores tend to sit as their body shapes change. However, anything that seems to be quite different to the norm – for example, a teenage boy who suddenly seems to acquire fat, rather than muscular thighs – is worth investigating.

What happens when you buy clothes for your child? Do you always have to purchase things two or three age sizes bigger because the waist will never do up, or the sleeves are always too tight? The waist in particular is a good guide because tall but slim children may need bigger age sizes because of their height, but in their case the waist invariably needs taking in to fit properly. This isn't a perfect

Girls waist circumference

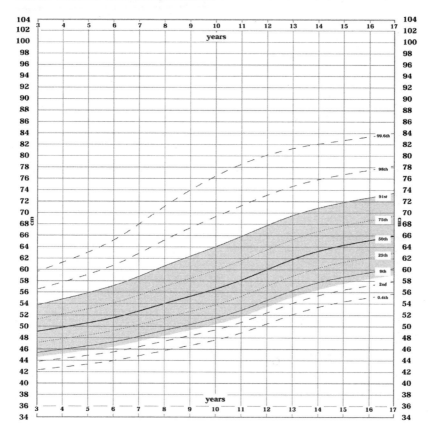

guide, however, as some younger children are simply bigger than the average, and still have the normal 'tummy' appropriate to their age, but you get the idea. It's also worth asking a couple of trusted friends for their opinion, but be careful to phrase the question in a way that allows them to answer honestly.

Remember, however, that children's shapes and fat distribution, as well as weight gain, change a great deal as they get older. Let's look at what is considered to be 'normal'.

Normal weight gain in children

From babyhood through to about five or six years of age, children accumulate more fat on their extremities than on their torsos. Then, proportionally more fat accumulates around the tummy and trunk until adolescence. And then it all goes mad! During the adolescent growth spurt, boys gain more fat on their trunks, while fat on their arms and legs decreases. Girls gain pretty much equal amounts of weight on their trunks and arms and legs during this period.

So the sudden appearance of a tummy after the age of six is not a sign of obesity, nor is this the case if your adolescent daughter suddenly develops more fat all over. In boys, the adolescent growth spurt means an obvious increase in weight, but this is principally bone tissue and skeletal muscle – and some fat. Girls, on the other hand, experience a slightly less intense spurt in height, a less obvious increase in skeletal muscle, but a continuous increase in fat mass. In girls the adolescent growth spurt starts around the age of nine or 10; in boys between 11 and 12, although this obviously varies between children.

On average, children gain around 2–3 kg (5–7 lb) per year between the ages of six and 10. As adolescence and puberty begin, growth rates increase, first in height and then in weight, although it is very normal for children to put on weight in advance of a major growth spurt. They fill out and then shoot up. Don't be alarmed at this. Girls tend to reach a peak growth period around 12 years of age, which then slows down until they are about 16 to 18. In their peak growth period (between the ages of 11 and 13), girls will put on about 7 kg (15 lb) in body weight – but it may be much more than this. In boys, the major growth spurt begins around 11 or 12, and reaches its maximum around the age of 14. Their growth rate then slows, but growth continues until they are about 18 to 20. During their peak growth period (between the ages of 13 and 15), boys gain an average of 14 kg (31 lb). Boys also tend to gain less fat than girls do during this period.

All in all, a child's body weight may double between the ages of 10 and 18. In boys the extra weight is mainly muscle; in girls the extra weight is muscle and also fat on hips and breasts, giving them a more rounded shape. It's important to distinguish womanly curves from fat – when your daughter enters adolescence, she will change shape so there is no need for concern unless the amount of weight gained is obviously more than it should be.

Children are all different, and they therefore mature and develop at different stages. Some are precocious and enter puberty

TOO MUCH FAT?

If you are in doubt about whether your child is carrying too much fat, your doctor should be your first port of call. If he or she thinks it necessary, the amount of fat your child has will be measured – usually by calculating waist measurement – and the figure compared to the standard for children of a similar age and height.

much earlier than others; some are late bloomers and do not experience a growth spurt until well into their mid teens. The message here is obviously to expect weight gain as part and parcel of other changes as your child grows up, but keep any eye on anything that seems out of the ordinary.

Fat and muscle

One of the reasons why children's weight shoots up so dramatically in adolescence is the fact that they develop more muscle. As you should by now be aware, muscle weighs significantly more than fat. The problem is that with current levels of inactivity amongst children – and increasingly sedentary lifestyles – kids are not developing as much muscle as they should. Therefore, they could actually be overweight, because expected levels of muscle have not developed, and they have put on too much fat in its place. That's one reason why it is important to use up-to-date growth charts. The researchers who developed the most recent charts are aware of the shift from muscle to fat and have taken it into consideration when working out normal and reasonable BMIs for children.

Looking at it from another point of view, however, a child who exercises a lot will have more muscle than fat and may be heavier than average. Again, look for consistency. A child who remains within his percentile, or close to it, and appears trim, does not have a weight problem – even if he does seem heavy for his age and height.

Eating habits and exercise

The way your child eats is not only a good determinant of whether he is likely to be overweight in future, but also a clue as to whether a weight problem is due to lifestyle factors, rather than something inherited or caused by a physical problem. Unhealthy eating patterns are undoubtedly the cause of most weight problems, and we'll look at this and other causes in more detail in the next chapter. If your child eats too much, eats compulsively or for emotional reasons, or simply eats unhealthy foods regularly, then they are likely to become overweight. The other main problem is exercise. If a child is inactive, no matter how little or well he eats, he's likely to experience weight problems at some point in the future. These lifestyle factors are crucial in determining potential weight problems, as well as making clear the reason for a sudden gain in weight. A child who suddenly puts on weight in adolescence may be due for a growth spurt, but if he eats unhealthily and gets little exercise, chances are that the weight gain is not due solely to natural development.

Have a look at the quiz below to see how your child fares. Although they may not have a weight problem now, an unhealthy lifestyle is a fairly certain determinant of an overweight future, and it may well explain a sudden gain in weight.

You'll notice that many of the questions relate to your own approach to food and your family's approach to healthy living in general. The reason for this is obvious: no child grows up in a vacuum and she will be strongly affected by the food and lifestyle choices you make for her. If your family never exercises, your children are unlikely to choose healthy leisure pastimes over regular family routine. If you comfort eat, or use food treats to soothe emotional upset, you are likely to instil in your child an association between food and comfort. If you constantly diet and then revert to unhealthy eating habits, are a faddy eater yourself, and do not serve healthy food as a matter of course, your children are unlikely to have habits that are any different. Children learn what they live, so make sure you establish healthy food and lifestyle habits for your child by setting a good example yourself.

Quiz

1 When it comes to school lunches, your child tends to eat:

A *Fast food – that's all that's available at school.*

B *A lunch packed at home that contains pre-packaged foods, such as*

white bread sandwiches, crisps, chocolate, sweets and a fizzy drink or
fruit 'drink' (as opposed to fresh fruit juice).
C *A lunch packed at home that contains foods such as tuna in a
wholemeal pita, baby carrots, fruit, yogurt and fruit juice, or a lunch
from the school lunchroom that's equally healthy.*

**2 When it comes to dinner in your household, at least four out of
seven days a week:**
A *Everyone tends to fend for themselves – you eat what you like when
you like.*
B *Everyone eats the same thing, but usually in front of the television.*
C *You eat together at the table, with the television off.*

**3 How many servings of fruits and vegetables do you include in
meals each day? (For information on servings, see pages 73–75.)**
A *Less than three.*
B *Three or four.*
C *Five or more.*

4 When you're feeling upset or depressed you:
A *Bake or buy treats for your children because it helps to take your mind
off your worries – or theirs.*
B *Indulge in a sweet treat, such as ice cream, biscuits or chocolate.*
C *Go for a long walk or bike ride, or even a drive to let off steam.*

**5 If your son's football team lost their match or your daughter
failed an exam and was very upset, what would you do?**
A *Buy or make a special treat – biscuits or pizza – and let them indulge.*
B *Allow them to sulk a little, talk it through and then promise to go out
for ice cream after dinner.*
C *Allow them to sulk a little then take them out with a friend to let off
some steam – by playing crazy golf, going for a bike ride, a swim or
some other activity.*

**6 How often do you allow your child to drink fizzy drinks or
sugary, fruit-based drinks (drinks that are less than 80 per cent
fruit juice)?**

A *Whenever she wants.*

B *With dinner most nights and on special occasions, such as birthdays or at the cinema.*

C *Very rarely.*

7 Your child is most likely to spend the three hours right after school:

A *Home alone, playing video games or watching TV while snacking on whatever he wants (typically fizzy drinks and crisps).*

B *Busy with an organized activity. On the days he's at home, he usually plays on the computer or games console with friends and has a healthy snack or a bowl of cereal.*

C *Most days he has an organized activity, or goes out on his bike or to the park with his friends. He has a piece of fruit or some cheese as a snack.*

8 Your doctor tells you that you are 11 kg (25 lb) overweight and that you need to lose weight for your health. You:

A *Ask about prescription diet pills or a quick method, because diets never work for you and you hate exercise.*

B *Know you should join a gym and try a diet programme like Weight Watchers, but find there's just not enough time in the day for exercise or attending the group meetings.*

C *Ask him for the name of a nutritionist or a good book on nutrition, to help you to change your eating habits. Promise yourself that you'll make an appointment at the gym, and that the whole family will begin to take regular walks after dinner and get some exercise at weekends.*

9 Your doctor tells you that your 12-year-old daughter is 4.5 kg (10 lb) overweight for her height. You:

A *Figure she'll keep growing and eventually it will even out.*

B *Start paying attention to everything she eats, and plan to give her a bicycle for her birthday.*

C *Work on changing family meals to include healthier options, and begin to make exercise a priority for the whole family.*

10 Which of the following most closely resembles a weekend with your family?

A *Staying in, eating takeaways, watching DVDs and playing video games; or going out to the local pizzeria or burger bar for dinner and then on to a film.*

B *Spending time working in the garden and doing household chores, then heading out to do some shopping, giving the kids treats or fast food while you're out.*

C *Planning day trips, such as cycling, hill-walking or a day of swimming and games on the beach, and then putting everyone to work in the kitchen afterwards to make homemade pizzas, a barbecue or a stir-fry for dinner.*

Interpreting the result

If most of your answers are As, you and your family are on target for weight problems. Substantial changes need to be made both to your leisure activities and your eating habits, which need to focus on nutritionally balanced meals and snacks. You need to recognize your role in instilling positive attitudes to fitness and food.

If most of your answers are Bs, you are halfway down the road to weight problems. Too much of your diet is centred around unhealthy food, or food for comfort, and leisure activities are not always healthy enough to keep overweight at bay. Make some simple changes, such as those outlined later in this book, to prevent weight from becoming an issue in your house.

If most of your answers are Cs, then keep on doing what you've been doing. Your overall attitude to meal planning, food behaviours and fitness in general indicate a reduced risk for raising an overweight or obese child. Activity and exercise are an integral part of your family life and, if you are concerned about your own weight, you understand the need to be proactive in order to maintain health. You also have a clear understanding of the importance of balanced meals and snacks.

Telltale signs of overeating

If your child has different eating patterns to you and the rest of your family, this may also be a cause for concern. Children who refuse to eat healthy foods, turn up their noses at fruit and vegetables, and demand sweets, crisps and fatty foods, are not likely to be getting the nutrients that they require to grow and develop properly, and they are also likely to be on the path to a weight problem. Similarly, children who eat secretly, stash away food in their rooms or 'steal' foods that are restricted, eat too quickly, always want second helpings or even just appear to eat much more than their peers may have issues about food that will affect their weight. Let's look at some of the danger signs.

Some children, very early on, become 'compulsive' eaters – something that is now considered to be a type of eating disorder. Uncontrollable eating and consequent weight gain characterize compulsive overeating. Compulsive overeaters tend to use food to cope with stress, emotional conflicts and daily problems. They may also overeat in response to an overly strict diet, either filling themselves up to avoid later feelings of hunger, as an act of rebellion against an overzealous carer or parent, or in order to satisfy a perceived need for foods that are not regularly offered. Children can be very clever about disguising compulsive overeating: they behave beautifully at home, eating only what is put in front of them, but later steal snacks, eat excessively when out of the house and binge on forbidden treats whenever possible. You may have come across this type of child yourself – overweight and with a parent who declares that she can't understand the problem because he doesn't overeat at home. However, when he's on his own, out of view of his parents, he eats far more and more quickly than anyone else and seems determined to get not just his share, but others as well – or stocks up on treats and sweets at every opportunity and eats them all in one go.

Compulsive overeating usually starts early in childhood when eating patterns are formed, but it can also develop in response to an overly strict diet, or because a child becomes the victim of abuse for being overweight and develops secretive habits and an unhealthy approach to food in general. Many children who become compulsive eaters never learned how to deal with a stressful situation other than through eating. Food can serve a protective function – it is something to hide behind and find comfort in. This is especially true of children who have been victims of some sort.

Some common signs of compulsive overeating include:
• Binge eating
• Not being able to stop voluntarily
• Withdrawing from activities due to being embarrassed by their weight
• Eating little in public, while continuing to put on weight or maintain overweight
• Eating little in the presence of parents, but bingeing or overeating when out of their sight
• Developing obsessions about food in general or different types of food, for example, having cravings for or aversions to specific foods
• Eating too quickly and too much
• Constant snacking, alongside regular meals.

There are also a number of other signs that your child is at risk of obesity and all the health and social problems associated with it. These include:

• Getting little exercise (less than 30 minutes per day)
• Choosing to play on the computer or games console, or watch television as the first choice of leisure activity
• Having an obese parent, or sibling
• Choosing fatty and junk foods when left to their own devices
• Eating fewer than the minimum recommended five servings of fruit and vegetables per day
• Snacking while watching television
• Eating more than 4 biscuits or a packet of crisps every day
• Drinking sugary soft drinks or fizzy drinks every day
• Being driven to and from school every day
• Spending more than 2 hours per day watching television
• Having few active interests
• Eating high-fat foods, such as crisps, chips, burgers and ice cream, more than five times per week
• Frequent snacks of junk food between meals
• Eating sweets every day.

While few of these factors alone is particularly damaging, if you can attribute more than two or three to your child, it's likely that poor habits are in place and that overweight and obesity will be the result. In later chapters we'll look at why each of these factors is important; for now, though, it's worth considering if your child's eating and lifestyle habits are putting him on course for problems.

What about fitness?

A whole chapter on fitness is included later in the book, but we can't overlook it here – because if your child is very unfit, does little or no exercise, and is unlikely to become involved in anything phys-ical without a substantial push, his weight will suffer. Young children are, by their nature, active and busy. Unfortunately, the advent of computer games, satellite TV, games consoles and the internet have put paid to physical activity for many children. Combine this with the often poor opportunities and facilities for exercise at school, and the fact that fewer families take part in healthy leisure activities together on a regular basis, and it's hardly surprising we are now seeing chil-dren who are dangerously inactive – even to the point of requiring a lift to and from school every day rather than walking a short dis-tance on their own.

Younger children seem to be able to do less exercise and not put on excess weight. They may get away with it, but that doesn't mean they are healthy, it simply means that they aren't showing the effects of a sedentary lifestyle – yet. Many younger children are care-fully fed healthy diets by their parents, but their activity levels are not monitored. And without both a good diet *and* reasonable exer-cise patterns in place, overweight can creep up and become a prob-lem later on. This is particularly common in pre-teenagers and ado-lescents, who are given freedom to make their own food choices for the first time, and tend to choose the same types of unhealthy foods that their friends are eating. If this is compounded by a sedentary lifestyle the weight will soon begin to pile on. So what your child does in her spare time is as important as what she eats in terms of preventing obesity – and dealing with it as a current problem. Your child might not yet be showing signs of overweight, but it's proba-bly on the cards if she's inactive.

So how fit is your child?

It's very easy to check a child's fitness levels. If your child is regularly active, you have no reason to worry. However, if you have a computer addict or bookworm in the house, their level of fitness may be inadequate. Watch your child for an average week and note down how long she spends being active. Answer the following questions and write down the number of points gained:

Quiz

Does your child:

1 Get some exercise (run, play actively, skip, jump or simply move around) for at least an hour a day?

add 2 points for every day (out of seven) that this occurs

2 Take part in school PE or games classes?

add 2 points for every session; subtract 1 point overall if classes are larger than 30 children

3 Take part in extracurricular sports activities such as tumble tots, swimming, gymnastics, football, cricket, ballet, dancing?

add 2 points for every hour spent at the activity

4 Attend classes, courses or activities where there is some physical activity involved (brownies, cub scouts, music and movement, etc.)?

add 2 points for every session

5 Choose physical activity above other hobbies or leisure activities on a regular basis?

add 1 point

6 Breathe heavily upon running up more than two flights of stairs (for children under the age of three, one flight of stairs)?

subtract 2 points

7 Continue to breathe heavily after a 10-minute break from high-exertion activities (in other words, breathing has not returned to normal after 10 minutes)?

subtract 2 points

8 Touch his or her toes easily?

subtract 2 points if they cannot

9 Spend more than 2 hours a day watching television, playing video or computer games, or reading?

subtract 2 points for every hour spent above 2 hours

10 Fall into the category of being obese (see page 3)?
subtract 2 points
11 Have less stamina than his peers (is able to run for less time,
finds keeping up difficult, etc.)?
subtract 2 points

Interpreting the result

Total your child's score.

Above 20 indicates a very high level of fitness – this child should
be in excellent condition. Unless food is a real problem, your child
should show no signs of overweight and, providing he keeps up
these habits into adulthood, he will remain a healthy weight.

A score of 14–19 reflects good exercise levels – this child should
be fit and able to keep up with or exceed the efforts of his peers.
Weight should not be a problem.

A score of 7–13 indicates a moderate degree of fitness – more
regular exercise would be beneficial and would reduce the child's
chances of becoming overweight.

Less than 7 equals unfit – try to find ways to increase exercise
levels, even if it's only slightly. If your child is not overweight now,
they are on course to be in the future.

In Chapter 5 we'll look at ways to fit exercise into your family
life, and to make it fun and appealing for children.

Using common sense

In this chapter we've looked at a variety of different ways of assessing whether or not your child is overweight – or at risk of becoming
so. With all the hype surrounding obesity, however, it is easy for parents to become alarmed about small changes in weight, and to try
to inflict diets upon children in an attempt to curb a trend. If you
think your child has a weight problem, don't panic. Stop and watch
her carefully for a month or two, to get an idea of her overall eating habits and activity levels. Work out if she's going through a
period of emotional difficulty that could be affecting her weight, or
if she's just entering a period of development where weight gain is
natural. If her weight continues to climb over this period, it's time
to take action. This book is designed to help parents deal with over-

weight in children in a way that preserves a child's self-esteem and allows them to develop healthy habits that they will carry with them into adulthood. There are no short-term solutions to weight prob-lems, as any adult dieter knows, and making drastic changes to your child's lifestyle and diet will probably rebound and cause problems that need not occur.

It's also important to look at the reasons why children gain weight. While it's obvious that eating too much and exercising too little will have an impact – and, indeed, these are the most common risk factors for overweight in children – there can be other reasons and it's worth investigating these before making any decisions or plans for dealing with the problem. Changing the eating habits of a child who is under pressure and using food for comfort is less likely to be successful than dealing with the stress that is causing the problem. Similarly, a faddy eater is unlikely to become a good eater overnight, so you have to work out an approach that gently eases your child into better eating habits. There may be blood sugar problems at the root, food allergies, or even genetic issues. Unless the causative fac-tors are addressed, any measures to get your child's weight under control are likely to have only short-term – if any – success.

The next chapter examines all the reasons why kids get fat, and helps you to assess your own child's particular problem.

Chapter Two

Why Kids Get Fat

Overweight children are often the target of abuse, typically because they are assumed to be lazy and to lack self-restraint. While it's pretty obvious that overeating, a poor diet and lack of exercise are the main reasons why children gain weight, it is important to take other factors into consideration, and to understand that our society has to take some of the blame for the lifestyle shifts that have led to the surge in obesity in both children and adults. No child sets out to be obese, or wilfully eats themselves to overweight. Nor do the majority of parents simply allow the problem to occur. There are other issues at the root of the growing trend towards obesity and it's important to examine these to get a clearer picture of why our children are becoming overweight.

Obesity is more common in broken families, in those with lower incomes and where one or both parents are poorly educated. It's easy, therefore, for many people to speculate that parents are to blame, and that ignorance, lack of money and dysfunctional family units underpin the problem. But the fact is that obese children now come from all types of backgrounds, classes and ethnic origins. Well-educated parents with plenty of money and a happy family unit also have overweight and obese children, as do very caring and switched-on families further down the income scale, so there is clearly more to the problem than income and education alone.

In this chapter we'll look at the various reasons why children put on weight, and become obese. In some cases it's a combination of factors that causes the problem and, indeed, the majority of overweight children have a set of unique characteristics that has led to weight gain. This means, of course, that apart from the obvious changes, such as increasing the level of exercise and encouraging a better diet, most parents will have to consider the distinct causative factors that apply to their individual child, and then adopt measures that are most suitable for him or her. The best way to do this is to read this chapter carefully, assess each of the issues in turn and then consider whether they are applicable to your child. Lifestyle factors can be fairly easily addressed and small changes to the way your family operates can also make a big difference. If emotional issues are at the root of your child's weight gain, then these too can be considered and addressed. Once again, the most important thing any parent can do is be realistic about the problem, take responsibility where required, and then deal sensitively with the matter in order to protect their child's self-esteem and self-image.

In this chapter there are several quizzes that are designed to help you pinpoint any physical or emotional problems that may be at the root of your child's weight gain, but the best assessment will be made if you are honest with yourself – and open to the idea that there may be things about your family's lifestyle that can be changed for the better. There may also be aspects of your child's lifestyle that may have eluded your attention and that can be adjusted to help ensure better health.

The modern child's diet

Until children are about six or seven, most parents have fairly close control over what their child eats. Therefore, the habits you put in place during this period can help to establish healthy eating patterns in the future, or at least instil in your child a very basic understanding of which foods are healthy. It sounds straightforward, but obviously there are other factors at play in determining what children choose to eat – and occasionally insist upon eating.

Despite what many parents try to achieve, the majority of our children eat too much junk. Even healthy diets are peppered with crisps, biscuits, sweets, cakes and fast food – the type of tempting treats that are aimed specifically at children. It takes a determined parent to resist the pleas of a child faced with an array of chocolates, chicken nuggets and chips in multi-coloured packaging, or sugar-coated cereals (complete with free toys) at the supermarket. It's also considerably easier to give in to a packet of sweets or to stop at a fast-food restaurant than it is to spend an afternoon bickering about it. It's not lack of education or even apathy that steers most parents in the wrong direction – it's usually exhaustion.

A diet based on junk

Even young children, whose parents make the majority of decisions regarding their diets, don't eat properly. According to the National Diet and Nutrition Survey in the UK, which was published in 2000, 70 per cent of preschoolers (children between the ages of 18 months and 4½ years) eat unhealthy foods such as biscuits, white bread, soft drinks, savoury snacks (including crisps and cereal-based snacks), chocolate, sweets and chips. The survey found that peas and carrots were the only cooked vegetables consumed by more than half the children surveyed, and of the 'vegetables', baked beans were consumed in the greatest quantities. Leafy green vegetables were eaten by only 39 per cent of the children and in fairly small quantities. And only 24 per cent ate raw vegetables or salad. Coated or fried fish was eaten by 38 per cent of the children surveyed, but white fish cooked by a method other than frying was eaten by only 10 per cent, while oily fish was eaten by just 16 per cent of the children. Some fruit appeared in the diets of most children, but it was limited mainly to apples, pears and bananas, while chocolate was consumed by 74 per cent of kids. Almost all had soft drinks (normally fizzy) and only a third of the children had fruit juice. Over 35 per cent of their diets were made up of fats and 29 per cent were sugars.

Regardless of how you look at it, this is not a healthy diet and it's no surprise that overweight is often the result. Foods that are high in salt, sugar and fat contribute to obesity and these appear to be the mainstay in the diets of many small children. And remember, these are children who are actually fed these foods rather than actively choosing or purchasing them for themselves.

What happens when dietary choices become more personal as they grow older? The same researchers looked at the diets of five- to 18-year-olds, with some even more alarming results. They found, for example, that 33 per cent of 15- to18-year-old girls smoke whereas only 20 per cent eat citrus fruits. Boys eat, by weight, nearly four times the amount of biscuits than they do leafy green vegetables. The most commonly consumed foods of the young people in the survey – eaten by over 80 per cent of the group – were white bread, savoury snacks, crisps, biscuits, boiled/mashed/jacket potatoes and chocolate confectionery. Over the seven-day recording period, less than 50 per cent of boys and 59 per cent of girls ate raw and salad vegetables, around 40 per cent ate cooked leafy green vegetables and 60 per cent ate other cooked vegetables, in comparison to the 88 per cent who ate chips. Carbonated soft drinks were the most popular beverage – 75 per cent of young people drank standard carbonated soft drinks and 45 per cent drank low calorie versions.

In the next chapter we'll look at what actually constitutes a healthy diet, but for now it's clear that the modern child's diet is at least partly to blame for the rise in overweight and obesity. Children are eating or being fed energy-dense food (food that is high in calories), such as sweets, crisps and chips, and not getting enough nutrient-dense foods, such as fruit and vegetables. The end result is, not surprisingly, unhealthy children with vitamin and mineral deficiencies and weight problems.

Empty tummies

A surprising number of children head off to school without breakfast (or at least anything recognizably nutritious). As a result their concentration suffers and they soon become genuinely hungry enough to seek out snacks – which, of course, are often poorly chosen and unhealthy (see page 32). Breakfast is a crucial meal when it comes to weight control. According to a 2003 study, published by the *American Journal of Epidemiology*, those who skip breakfast have a 4.5 times greater risk of obesity than those who eat breakfast regularly. 'Our results suggest that breakfast may really be the most important meal of the day,' says researcher Mark A. Pereira, PhD.

According to Pereira, eating breakfast might have beneficial effects on appetite, insulin resistance and energy metabolism: 'Just the habit of filling your belly in the morning might help people control their hunger throughout the day so they might be less likely to overeat in the morning or at lunch'.

Unfortunately, many children tend to skip breakfast and fill up on energy drinks or chocolate instead. One survey of nine- to16-year-olds found that the average child skips breakfast entirely 17 mornings out of 100 – and often relies on snack food on other occasions.

Regular meals

Breakfast isn't the only meal to be falling out of favour in our 24/7 culture, where kids are often rushed from activity to activity without a proper meal, or parents return home too late to provide one. All too often families develop a 'fend for yourself' mentality that results in even young children making their own food choices and eating whenever they like – and often alone, in front of the television.

Many children eat on the run, and unhealthy snacks form the basis of their daily diets. Eating out is increasingly common – a 2001 study showed that 75 per cent of students surveyed had eaten in a fast-food restaurant at least once in the previous week. The frequency with which students ate at these restaurants was related to an increase in total calories (mainly from fat), and consumption of soft drinks, burgers, chips and pizza, and inversely related to daily

VENDING MACHINES

These are the bane of parents and healthcare experts alike. No matter how hard we work to get the healthy eating message across, when children are faced daily with tempting treats, all for the cost of a little pocket money, they are unlikely to make the right choices. Vending machines undermine our efforts to teach our children to eat well, encouraging them to fill up on snacks that they simply don't need. In the UK and the US, these machines have been the subject of intense debate, and many companies providing the machines to schools in particular have promised to supply fruit juice, water and healthier snacks alongside confectionery and fizzy drinks. But how many kids are likely to actually choose the healthier options, given peer pressure, the impact of advertising and the tempting nature of unhealthy snacks? Not many. Vending machines are part of the snack culture and for some children their contents make up their entire lunch and even breakfast – little wonder then that obesity is on the increase.

servings of fruit, vegetables and milk. In other words, these kids were filling up on junk at the expense of healthier foods, hence their levels of calcium, fibre, vitamin A, vitamin C and beta-carotene – all crucial vitamins and minerals for growth and development – were lower. Teenagers who had visited fast-food outlets three or more times in the week preceding the study were significantly more likely to report that healthy foods tasted 'bad', and that they lacked the time to eat healthy foods.

The reality is that many children simply have no experience of 'healthy' meals and in comparison with the salt-, sugar- and fat-laden foods that regularly form the basis of their diets, healthy alternatives seem bland and unappetizing. It's a dangerous cycle, and children begin to demand the equivalent of fast food for all of their meals; a request that busy parents often give in to in order to ensure that their children are eating something at home. The problem is, of course, that children who are given unhealthy, fatty foods develop a taste for them. Hence fatter children tend to prefer high-fat foods, consume higher-fat diets and have parents with the highest BMI (body mass index). So fatter kids are, not surprisingly, eating fattier foods. Whether this causes the problem or exacerbates it is not clear, but chances are that if your child has a high-fat diet, he's on course to becoming overweight – if he isn't already.

Obviously today's society has something to do with the decline in good eating habits. The number of families who regularly eat dinner together has decreased enormously. Today, only one-third of families are estimated to dine together daily. An immediate effect of the decline in family meals is that children are spending more time eating outside the home. You'll find more on this on page 53, How Much Time Do You Spend With Your Children?

According to research from Cancer Research UK, the most influential aspect of a young child's environment is the family, and parental eating habits are an important part of this. Their research has suggested that parents can influence their children's eating habits by controlling mealtime routines. Regular family meals are related to healthier dietary patterns and a higher intake of fruit and vegetables in older children – and not surprisingly, children who eat more fruit and vegetables tend to have fewer problems with weight.

School lunches

Despite initiatives to improve the content of school meals, much of the fare on offer is heavily laden with fat, salt and sugar – largely because this is what children demand and, in some cases, the only thing they claim to eat. As we noted earlier, too, vending machines tempt children away from the lunch counter and encourage them to eat unhealthy snacks in place of a good meal. Many parents assume that their kids have had a good lunch, so often feel justified in cutting corners at home. Still more parents are largely unaware of what their children are eating during the day, and fail to realize that chips form the basis of most children's lunch – every single day. Combined with snacks purchased on the way home from school, many kids are simply not hungry for nourishing meals prepared at home, having filled up on junk all day long.

Unhealthy snacking

To meet energy needs, children and teenagers should eat at least three meals a day, beginning with breakfast. Snacks should also form an integral part of their meal patterns. Young children in particular cannot eat large quantities of food at one sitting and get hungry long before the next regular mealtime. Mid-morning and mid-afternoon snacks serve an important purpose – keeping blood sugar levels stable, supplying important nutrients and providing the energy that children need to be active. But the key thing to remember is that snacks must be healthy, as they contribute to your child's overall health and nutritional status.

FAST-FOOD PORTIONS

Portion sizes are steadily increasing for both ready-to-eat and restaurant meals. In many fast-food restaurants, a single 'super-sized' or 'extra-value' meal provides more than an entire day's worth of calories. Unfortunately, almost a third of the population base the amount of food they eat on how much food is on their plates; and for these people, growing portion sizes can easily contribute to growing waistlines.

If you don't provide your child with appropriate snacks, chances are she'll seek them out herself and make unsuitable choices. In the UK, children spent £433 million on sweets, crisps and fizzy drinks on their journeys to and from school in 2002, according to the Sodexho School Meals and Lifestyle Survey. This was up from £365 million in 2000. In 2000, *The Times* published a survey of 1390 children, which found that the average child spends £6 per week on sweets, crisps and fizzy drinks. This represented a rise of 40 per cent on the previous survey, undertaken just two years earlier. These purchases were often made in newsagents and shops where a range of healthy options was available. In addition, only two per cent of children purchased water either on their way to school or on their journey home. If fruit or healthy snacks were purchased, their consumption was too low to be registered in the survey.

There's also plenty of evidence that a great deal of snacking takes place in front of the television (see page 58), and this obviously has an impact on weight.

The soft drink culture

Soft drinks are everywhere and the peer pressure exerted on our children to drink them is enormous. These drinks are a real problem, but one that many parents overlook. A 2002 study discovered that children who drink more sweetened beverages, such as fizzy drinks, sweetened juices and high-calorie drinks, have an overall higher calorie intake (an average of 330 calories a day, or about one-fifth of the calorie intake recommended for a whole day), are less likely to eat fruit (62 per cent less fruit than those who drank fewer sweetened drinks) and are at a higher risk of obesity.

And the problem is growing. More than 60 per cent of all pupils in the UK now drink one can a day, and one in six drinks a staggering 22 cans a week. The intake of fizzy drinks and sweetened non- or low-fruit juices has increased by more than 900 per cent over the last 40 years. And since 1978, soft drink consumption has risen dramatically, with intake doubling in children aged six to 11 and tripling amongst teenage boys.

Currently, soft drinks constitute the leading source of added sugars in the diet and the levels of consumption often approach or exceed the recommended daily limits for *total* added sugar consumption. And sugar has a real impact when it comes to weight problems (see page 35). Significantly, the dramatic rise in soft drink consumption coincides almost exactly with the significant increase in childhood and adolescent obesity.

Cutting out the fizzy or sugary drinks could make a big difference. Interestingly, it's not necessarily the calories causing the problem. Research into sugar substitutes (artificial sweeteners) has found that they are as detrimental to weight as sugar.

Too much fat

It goes without saying that if you eat too much fat some will be laid down as fat, and cause weight gain. We've looked at the fact that so much of the food that children eat today is laden with fat, which has caused them to develop a taste for fatty fare, but it can be argued that too much emphasis has been placed on the *amount* of fat in the diet as the main cause of weight problems. Certainly it is one cause, but it is certainly not the only one. In fact, some studies claim that there is no real link between the amount of fat consumed and a child's weight, which means that an over focus on the quantity of fat in your child's diet may be irrelevant.

While it may be difficult to believe that there is no link, consider the fact that low- and no-fat products have become increasingly popular over the last five years or so – and many families have changed their eating habits to incorporate such foods – yet obesity levels have continued to increase. Low-fat products are not the godsend their producers would have us believe. Not only do low-fat products tend to have many more chemicals included in their makeup, in order to make them palatable, some of them are downright dangerous (see Trans Fats page 76). Most importantly, perhaps, healthy eating habits are never learned if children grow up eating lower-fat versions of unhealthy foods. Crisps, cakes, sweets, chips, chicken nuggets and other such so-called 'kiddie' foods are as unhealthy when they are low in fat as they are when they contain their normal level of fat. If a child never learns another way of eating, he's not going to develop the healthy eating habits necessary to maintain a reasonable weight.

It's the *type* of fat your child eats that is most important. If your child eats too many trans fats, commonly found in commercial baked goods and fast foods, he'll be at higher risk of cardiovascular disease and type 2 diabetes. At the opposite end of the spectrum, fats found in vegetables and their oils, as well as fish and seafood, tend to reduce the risks. And it's the health problems associated with fat that are most worrying.

Fat is a necessary part of a healthy diet, so going overboard by removing it from your child's diet, or switching to low-fat products, may backfire. Indeed, removing fat from your child's diet might lead to cravings and nutritional deficiencies. The secret is to ensure your child gets an adequate amount of the healthier fats and fewer of the unhealthy sources of fat. In the next chapter we'll look at the different kinds of fat and how healthy or damaging they are.

What about carbs?

This is a source of real confusion for parents – and I'm not surprised. About a decade ago, fat was labelled the big 'baddie' and people were encouraged to change their diets to include lots more carbohydrates (rice, bread products, baked goods, for example). But did the level of overweight and obesity go down? No. In fact, the opposite appears to be true. And that's largely because the increased level of carbohydrates in our diets has come in the form of refined foods such as breads, pastas, processed cereals, potatoes, soft drinks, cakes and biscuits. Many carbohydrate products are adapted to have 'no fat', so anyone worried about their weight may think, hey, the perfect way to fill up without taking in too much fat. But it goes without saying that most of these foods are not particularly nutritious. The over-emphasis on losing fat from our diets has meant that instead of changing the way we eat to include healthier foods, we've focused instead on filling up on anything that is fat-free. Ironically that hasn't meant an increase in the consumption of fresh, fat-free fruit and vegetables. Instead, it has led to people eating yet more junk, which is presumed to be acceptable because the fat levels are lower.

But then came the Atkins diet and carbs became taboo again. So what exactly is the problem with carbohydrates? First of all, many have a high glycaemic index, or GI (which we will discuss in more detail in the following chapter), which basically means that they cause fairly large increases in blood sugar levels after they are eaten. And, if you eat too much sugar it will be laid down as fat – just as too much fat is laid down as fat – because the body simply cannot use up all the energy it provides. However, it's a little more complicated than that.

Consuming meals composed of predominantly high-GI foods causes a sequence of hormonal events in your child's body that stimulate hunger and cause overeating (particularly in adolescents). Perhaps more worrying is that a high-GI diet may actually do as much damage to your child's health as a diet that's high in saturated fat. A high-GI diet has been linked with obesity, cardiovascular disease and type 2 diabetes – the very problems that switching from fat to carbohydrates is supposed to prevent!

There is a way round this conundrum and that is to choose foods for your children that have a low GI. Low GI foods, such as wholegrains, brown rice, wholewheat pasta, wholegrain breakfast cereals and many fruits and vegetables, have the opposite effect of high-GI foods, and, what's more, studies show that these types of foods seem to positively influence the feeling of being full, and reduce the need or desire to eat more. So carbohydrates are, like fat, definitely on the menu, but again you need to look at the *type* of carbohydrates you are serving. You'll find more on this in the next chapter.

For now, it's fair to say that if your child's diet is heavily weighted in favour of carbohydrates with a high GI (the majority of foods that kids love) it's a likely cause of their weight problem.

Sugar
Sugar is pretty closely tied in with the blood sugar problems associated with high-GI carbohydrates. In fact, sugar is pretty much pure carbohydrate – of the very worst kind. Many parents worry about sugar in their children's diets because it decays their teeth, and also because it tends to make them overactive and difficult to deal with. But, because it contains no fat, it tends to get overlooked as a cause of obesity.

However, sugar plays a crucial role in weight gain, and here's why. When it is a natural part of food, sugar is not particularly problematic. Most foods contain some natural sugars and when they are digested as part of a 'whole' food (for example, fruit, vegetables or unprocessed grains) they don't tend to send blood sugar levels soaring in the same way that pure sugars do. The problem with sugar lies in the fact that we have learned to extract the sweetness of foods and concentrate it. These types of sugars, such as white sugar, brown sugar, glucose, honey, syrup, malt and so on, are 'fast-releasing', which means that they cause blood sugar levels to go sky high – and, of course, sugar which is not required by the body is stored and eventually laid down as fat. We all know that too many calories cause weight gain, but these types of sugars have also normally been stripped of vitamins and minerals, so they effectively provide 'empty' calories to boot!

It doesn't take long to check the packaging on a few of your child's favourite foods. Most will contain sugars, and pretty high levels of them. Add to that the amount of high-sugar soft drinks the average child consumes, and you can see how their intake soars. High blood sugar is one of the main causes of overweight in children. This is discussed in more detail on page 40.

Imbalances and other physical causes

It's clear to see that the modern child's diet is at the very least partly to blame for the rise in the incidence of overweight and obesity, and their eating habits undoubtedly contribute to the trend. However, there are also other factors that can affect your child's weight, and some of these have to do with your child's overall health. It's a bit of a chicken and egg situation – many of the problems that may underpin a weight problem are caused by an unhealthy diet in the first place, but once they are in place, they exacerbate the problem and create cravings for more unhealthy food. So if you do discover that there is a physical cause behind your child's weight problem, you may find that addressing his diet will have a big impact on his weight and overall health.

Dieting

The focus on weight has meant that many children are on strict diets from an early age – either because they are put on one by overzealous parents, or because kids insist on it themselves because they perceive themselves to be fat. Our culture is partly to blame for this – girls all want to be stick-thin, like their media heroes, and boys want to have the lithe, toned bodies of athletes and boy band stars. Surveys of teenagers in the UK consistently show greater than 50 per cent of girls feel fat and want to lose weight and about 20 per cent of boys the same age are similarly dissatisfied. In the natural course of growing up, a few pounds are gained here and there. However, if this is perceived to be 'fat' and parents or the children themselves become aghast, it's all too easy for them to develop an inaccurate body image and start to monitor their diets. Ironically, of course, this tendency to diet at increasingly younger ages has not led to a reduction in weight overall – it has coincided with the biggest surge in obesity in living memory.

Why is this? Well, as any adult dieter can tell you, diets simply don't work. Just about any diet will work for a while because it disrupts the individual's usual eating pattern. Whether the dieter eats grapefruits with every meal or goes on a high-fat low-carbohydrate diet, the intense effort at dieting, coupled with water loss, results in an initial success that boosts self-esteem and provides further motivation – but bizarre diets can't be continued for a lifetime and should never be considered safe for growing children. Unusual diets and crash diets are doomed to failure because anyone with a weight problem can't depend on their own appetite to control their weight, and therefore needs to learn new eating habits that they can depend on for the rest of their life. Furthermore, when a child tries to make their body thinner than it is genetically programmed to be, it retaliates by becoming ravenous and vulnerable to binge eating. Ninety-eight per cent of dieters regain all the weight they manage to lose, plus about 10 extra pounds, within five years. Hence, yo-yo dieting results in a cycle of weight loss followed by ever-increasing weight gain, as hunger repeatedly wins.

Much debate centres around the dangers and benefits of dieting in children and adolescents. In one aspect dieting at an early age is central to eating disorders and has a strong association with extreme weight control and unhealthy behaviours. One study found that, in the long run, early dieting and excessive exercise regimes aimed at weight loss may be associated with the development of chronic body image problems, weight cycling (when weight rises and falls on a consistent basis), eating disorders and obesity. It seems that parents play a detrimental role when they create an environment that emphasizes thinness and dieting, or excessive exercise, as a way to attain the desired body. In addition, commenting on a child's weight or body shape – which tends to become more common as children get older – can have a strong influence on children, who may develop a negative self-image, an obsession with thinness and an equally obsessional way of dealing with perceived weight problems.

Very recent research has also pointed to the inefficiency of diets. Researchers at Brigham and Women's Hospital have found that boys and girls who diet to lose or maintain weight may actually be doing the reverse. The research found that although children who said they were dieters reported being more active and eating fewer

 CASE HISTORY: Elizabeth

A slim child, Elizabeth experienced puberty in advance of many of her friends, and had her growth spurt early as well. She was big-boned and while she was not considered remotely fat by her family or friends, she hated being larger and more developed than her peers so put herself on a strict diet. She lost weight initially, but soon developed an unhealthy relationship with food – starving herself and over-exercising, then succumbing to temptation and bingeing for days on end. Her weight eventually began to rise beyond normal levels, which compounded her fear that she was 'different' from her peers. It wasn't until her friends began to experience the normal gains of weight associated with puberty, and to develop more womanly curves, that she felt she fitted in. Unfortunately, by this time, her weight had become a real problem. Although Elizabeth had been within normal bounds for her age and build, she developed a negative body image that eventually sent her weight rocketing. Had she been made to feel 'normal' and taught that puberty changes bodies and that builds differ between children, she may not have felt so isolated.

calories than their peers, they gained more weight than non-dieters. For example, a 14-year-old girl who was a frequent dieter gained about 1 kg (2 lb) per year more than other 14-year-old girls who did not diet. Girls who dieted less often gained slightly less weight, but still significantly more than non-dieters. 'At a time when we need solutions to encourage healthy eating habits, it is troubling to see that dieting, which is often characterized by short-term and not necessarily healthy changes in eating, is so common,' noted researcher Alison Field. 'Our study found that dieting was counterproductive – children who dieted gained more, not less, weight than non-dieters.'

Field and her team provided several possible explanations for the link. The most likely is that dieting may lead to a cycle of restrictive eating, followed by bouts of overeating or binge eating. The repeated cycles of overeating, between the restrictive diets, may be responsible for weight gain. The fact that dieters were more likely to binge-eat than their non-dieting peers supports this hypothesis.

When the researchers studied the mothers of these children, they found that the behaviours or lifestyle factors associated with weight control, or lack thereof, were established by late adolescence. However, this latest research suggests that dieting behaviours may manifest at a much younger age

If your child is a regular dieter, this may well be contributing to her problem.

Nutritional deficiencies

The poor diets of many children have left them undernourished – a great tragedy given the amount of good, healthy food that is available. To make matters worse, nutritional deficiencies can also contribute to overweight. If your child eats a diet similar to that mentioned earlier – lots of fast, junk or convenience foods, too much sugar, unhealthy fats and too many soft drinks – he's likely to be deficient in many of the key nutrients. One study found that the majority of preschoolers had vitamin and mineral intakes far below recommended levels. A case in point is iron, which is required for growth, the production of haemoglobin (the part of the blood that carries oxygen) and certain enzymes, immunity and energy. Eighty-four per cent of those under four years of age and 57 per cent of those aged four and four and a half had intakes below the lowest recommended levels. Older children didn't fare any better. Without good levels of iron, children feel tired and lack energy, which leads to cravings for sweet foods and other pick-me-ups, such as caffeine. The upshot of this, of course, is that children who lack energy are unlikely to feel like exercise. So it's a bit of a double whammy.

Our bodies are like intricate machines and they require fuel to keep them working effectively. If the fuel is missing some key components, then things start to go wrong. The fine balance of our body chemistry is upset and health problems can be the result. And it is these health problems that can lead, or at least contribute, to overweight. For example, the mineral chromium is often missing in the diets of modern children, and this affects the way their bodies deal with sugar. Cravings are often the result of this deficiency. Other nutrients affect metabolism and even mood, which has an impact on the way children view themselves and the food choices they make.

If your child's diet is poor, he may be missing some key nutrients from his diet – nutrients that affect his health and weight.

Blood sugar problems

Closely linked to obesity and a whole host of other health and emotional problems is an issue we've already touched on briefly – the issue of blood sugar imbalance. This is a big problem for many children these days, largely because their diets are so high in sugar and refined carbohydrates.

Every moment of every day, the body adjusts its internal mechanisms to keep itself in balance. The name given to this principle of internal balance is 'homeostasis'. One very important component of homeostasis is the regulation of the level of sugar in the bloodstream. However, the mechanisms that are designed to keep blood sugar on an even keel can fail. In the short term, an imbalance in the blood sugar level can give rise to symptoms such as fluctuating energy, mood swings and cravings for sweet and starchy foods. In the long term, problems such as weight gain, high cholesterol and diabetes can arise too.

For most children, and probably the majority of adults, a significant proportion of their diet comes in the form of carbohydrates

– for example fruit, fruit juices, confectionery, cakes, biscuits, bread, potatoes, rice, pasta and cereals. When we eat carbohydrates our blood sugar level rises. When this happens, a hormone called insulin is secreted by the pancreas. One of the chief purposes of insulin is to transport sugar out of the bloodstream and store it in the body's cells to provide energy. In this way, blood sugar is lowered again, preventing the accumulation of sugar in the bloodstream (which eventually leads to diabetes). As I pointed out earlier, the body copes well with foods which release sugar relatively slowly into the bloodstream. However, if the blood sugar level rises very quickly, the body tends to secrete a lot of insulin in response. The problem here is that this drives blood sugar levels lower than normal, a condition which is referred to as 'hypoglycaemia'. Hypoglycaemia has a whole host of symptoms, including:

- Fatigue. This is usually experienced as peaks and troughs of energy as the blood sugar levels rise and fall.

- Mid-afternoon sleepiness or lack of concentration. The rise in blood sugar following lunch (which can be particularly dramatic if your child has eaten sweets, drunk fizzy drinks, or had refined carbs) can cause insulin to surge, leading to low blood sugar and sleepiness later.

- Morning grogginess. This is something that many parents will recognize. The fatigue associated with hypoglycaemia is often at its worst first thing in the morning. Children prone to blood sugar imbalances tend not to maintain blood sugar levels unless they eat. For this reason, blood sugar can fall during the night, leading to fatigue and grogginess in the morning.

- Generally poor concentration, low mood or irritability. Although the brain makes up only about two per cent of our weight, at rest it uses roughly half the sugar circulating in our bloodstream. What's more, while most of the body can use other foods to generate energy, the brain is almost entirely reliant on sugar for normal and healthy functioning.

- Night waking. When blood sugar levels drop during the night, your child's body may attempt to correct this by secreting hormones that stimulate the release of sugar from the liver. The main hormone that the body uses for this is adrenalin, which increases arousal and may trigger feelings of anxiety and even panic. Therefore, blood sugar problems can cause your child to wake in the night, and can even cause nightmares.

- Food cravings. When your child's blood sugar level drops it is natural for her body to crave foods it knows will restore the blood sugar level quickly. This commonly manifests as cravings for sweet and/or starchy foods.

Does all this sound familiar? The symptoms of blood sugar imbalance are most obvious when sugar levels are low. However, the excess insulin the body secretes to keep blood sugar in check, can itself cause serious problems. The effects of excess insulin include:
- Fat production
- High blood pressure and fluid retention
- Raised cholesterol
- Type 2 diabetes

And this is when it becomes even more serious. Fifty per cent of people diagnosed with type 2 diabetes have significant cardiovascular disease at the time of diagnosis. And 80 per cent of diabetic deaths are due to cardiovascular disease. Obesity has been directly linked to the onset of type 2 diabetes, a disease that usually hits people in their 30s or 40s. But with one in five children now said to be overweight, some studies indicate the number of young people with type 2 diabetes has quadrupled in recent years.

Puberty has been identified as an important stage in the development of type 2 diabetes in children. Changes in hormone levels during this period can cause problems with the way the body deals with insulin, hence many cases of type 2 diabetes rear their heads in puberty. But the worrying thing is that kids as young as four have been diagnosed with type 2 diabetes.

Obesity is another significant factor. Obese children produce too much insulin, because their body cells have been so flooded with insulin for so long that they lose their sensitivity to it, hence the body must produce more for it to be effective. This causes the cells to become even more resistant to insulin. In this situation, the blood insulin levels are chronically higher, which inhibits the fat cells from giving up their energy stores to allow weight loss. This is because the body concludes that the presence of insulin indicates that there is adequate blood sugar available to provide energy and therefore there is no need for the release of fats from fat tissue.

If your child suffers from any of the symptoms outlined on pages 41–42, blood sugar problems may well be part of the problem. A sensitivity to sugar and refined carbohydrates is increasingly common in kids today, and it's clear to see that this can have a dramatic effect on both weight gain and potential weight loss.

Food sensitivities

Food allergies and intolerances are on the increase, for reasons that are not clearly understood. What we do know, however, is that these sensitivities can affect digestion, lead to cravings, cause bloating and mood swings, and create a feeling of fatigue. If your child is suffering from a sensitivity, he may feel lethargic and unable to rouse himself to do anything active; he may crave the same foods over and over again, and he may feel depressed, anxious or moody, and feel the need for comfort foods to feel better.

A food intolerance is an adverse reaction caused by specific foods. For example, lactose intolerance occurs when the sufferer lacks an enzyme that is needed to digest milk sugar. When that child (or adult) eats milk products, she will experience symptoms such as wind, bloating, diarrhoea and/or abdominal pain. A sensitivity is simply a milder reaction, and the symptoms are not normally as dramatic.

Interestingly, research shows that it is almost always the most commonly eaten foods that are the source of the problem. In Britain and other Western countries, wheat and milk are key culprits, largely because they are consumed several times every day. Research into this is on-going but it seems that a large intake of any food, regardless of what it is, can trigger off an intolerance to that food. The body appears to become overloaded and develops a mild resistance to the food as a sort of self-protection measure.

Symptoms are often difficult to pinpoint, largely because they can seem innocuous in the early stages. The time it takes for symptoms to appear can also make it harder to link a reaction with a specific food. Some children become intolerant after a course of antibiotics, or being exposed to pesticides or other toxins. Symptoms may become worse in periods of stress, or after illness, which also clouds the issue. Some of the most common symptoms include:

- anxiety
- asthma
- bedwetting in children over the age of three or four (although this has other causes)
- behavioural problems
- bloating
- chronic sniffling
- constipation
- coughing
- Crohn's disease
- diarrhoea
- eczema
- excess mucus
- facial puffiness
- fatigue
- flatulence
- headaches
- hives
- IBS
- indigestion
- insomnia
- itchy eyes
- itchy skin
- mood swings
- mouth ulcers
- muscular aches
- nausea
- skin rashes (around the mouth, particularly, although the whole body may be affected)
- sore throats
- water retention
- wheezing

The best way to test for intolerance is to look for any changes in your child's health, even if it has been a slow progressive change. Does your child complain of headaches or excessive fatigue after meals? Does he get inexplicable skin rashes, particularly around his mouth? Is his behaviour worse after a particular type of food? Does he crave a particular type of food constantly? This is a strange feature of food intolerance, and it may be something that you have noticed in your own diet. There is plenty of evidence to suggest that we crave the foods to which we are intolerant. Some studies show that at least 50 per cent of us suffer food cravings for problem foods. We may even be unaware of it. Look at the foods your child chooses,

particularly if she is a picky eater. Children who refuse to eat anything other than pasta, cereal and bread, show clear-cut tendencies
for suspect foods. You may find that cravings and aversion are affecting normal healthy eating patterns and these are, in turn, affecting
your child's weight.

Metabolism

Some overweight adults blame their problem on a 'slow metabolism',
and claim to have inherited this type of disorder. First of all, metabolism does obviously affect weight, as it dictates the rate at which
you burn calories to turn them into energy. Some children do have
slower metabolisms than others, but this is not as serious as it sounds.
For example, how much your child eats, when he eats and whether
or not he skips meals can affect his metabolism. If he eats a snack
instead of a proper dinner, and regularly misses breakfast, his body
will think it is 'starving' and slow down the rate at which it burns
calories – a kind of survival tactic. This means that the meals he eats
during the day will be less efficiently processed because his metabolism is slower than it should be. Another factor affecting metabolism is exercise. Exercise, very simply, speeds up metabolism, as the
body requires more energy to keep going. So a sluggish metabolism
could simply be due to the fact that meals are not regular, and your
child is not getting enough exercise.

Hereditary factors can also influence a child's metabolism. It is
known that a child's weight is most closely correlated with that of
its mother. And if you have a sluggish or an efficient metabolism yourself, as a mother, the chances are your children will inherit much the
same. But remember, children with a slow metabolism can speed it
up with exercise and regular meals; those with an efficient metabolism simply have to learn to eat less, and usually smaller, more frequent meals will keep a potential problem under control.

Hormones

A small minority of cases of obesity can be explained by glandular
or hormonal problems. One such problem is clinical hypothyroidism,
where there is not enough thyroid hormone to control normal rates
of metabolism. This is very rare in children, but those who are very

obese may need to have their thyroid gland function checked by a specialist. Another hormone-related disorder that can cause overweight is Cushing's syndrome, a rare condition caused by excess corticosteroid hormones in the body. Again, this is a problem that needs to be addressed by a doctor, and usually only when other weight loss methods have failed, and there is a clear indication of symptoms. A variety of hormonal disorders, including problems with insulin, hypothalamic hormones and pituitary hormones, can cause severe obesity. There are also a number of rare inherited syndromes (such as Laurence-Moon-Biedl and Prader-Willi) that produce obesity. If a child's height is appropriate or advanced for her age, one of these underlying medical conditions is extremely unlikely. On the other hand, an obese child with slow height growth should certainly be evaluated for any such problem.

Sex hormones can also affect obesity. In girls, body fat levels during adolescence are determined by the balance of female sex hormones. Changes in energy intake, desire for food and specific cravings also occur at various stages of the menstrual cycle. Some girls appear to be more susceptible than others to hormonal changes. If your daughter's weight problems started around puberty, she may have a hormonal imbalance or a sensitivity to the effect of hormones and this can often be treated.

In addition, hormones produced when we are under stress encourage the formation of fat cells. In Westernized countries, life tends to be competitive, fast-paced, demanding and stressful – even for children. In fact, stress is a growing problem in today's kids (we'll look at this in the following pages) and there may be a link between so-called modern life and increasing rates of overeating, overweight and obesity.

Genetics

Like metabolism, certain aspects of physiology can be inherited from parents, and your child may have a genetic disposition to overweight. When one parent is obese there is a 25–30 per cent risk that their children will be obese. This risk increases to up to 80 per cent when both parents are obese. Some of this is obviously down to lifestyle and habits – which children acquire and consider normal – but there is also evidence that a tendency to fat is inherited as well. Some studies suggest that genetic factors account for 25–40 per cent of obesity cases. Other studies put the figure closer to 5–25 per cent. Regardless of which is the more accurate, the relationship between genetics and your child's environment is clear: parents provide genes, role models and food.

Some studies show that the way that fat is distributed on your child's body can be inherited. Body shape, for example, generally falls into three categories – ectomorph, endomorph and mesomorph. Ectomorphs have slight frames and a low capacity for storing fat, while endomorphs have the most fat storage capacity. Mesomorphs have an ability to store fat somewhere in between – and it tends to be pretty evenly distributed. So if you have a heavy build that your child has inherited, he will have a predetermined disposition to store fat in a certain way. However, storing fat in excess is quite another matter, and body shape and fat distribution are unlikely to be enough to cause obesity. There must be other factors – such as diet and lifestyle – at work.

This does bring up an interesting question, though. Children with a bigger build, and a disposition to store more fat, might feel larger than their slighter peers, and consider themselves to be 'fat' or 'overweight' when they aren't. This can lead to all the negative feelings associated with overweight (see page 48), and actually exacerbate the problem or even create one.

There's no doubt that genes do make a difference to your child's shape and body weight. If a child is chubby but eats healthily, exercises regularly, does not have any emotional factors affecting the way he eats, he may just be genetically predisposed to be heavier than average. Research suggests that this kind of extra weight is not as much of a health risk as the kind acquired by eating too many unhealthy snack foods and too many hours sitting in front of a TV or computer. Genetically podgy children may be healthier chubby than if they are forced to diet to fit in with slim peers.

Whatever your child's genetic make-up, it's important to remember that childhood obesity is a modern phenomenon – certainly one that has become much more common over the last five to 30 years. While evolution can cause a population's gene pool to shift, this occurs over billions of years – certainly not a few decades. The gene pool of humans has not changed much over the last 30 years in which fat has become a problem. Therefore, there is no new 'obesity' gene to blame for the problem. Genes can affect the weight of some children, but it isn't the main cause of this dangerous trend.

Emotional factors

There is a great deal of evidence that emotional health underpins at least part of the trend towards obesity, and this is something that parents simply may not have considered relevant. Like adults, children often rely on 'food fixes' to deal with emotions. They eat more when they are feeling sad, stressed or bored, and they are particularly likely to do so if their parents do this.

Again, this is a problem that is two-fold. Children who put on weight for one of any variety of reasons, begin to lose their self-esteem. Part of the reason for this is the fact that overweight children are stereotyped. A 1995 study, for example, found that even nine-year-old children considered overweight children to be:

• Unhealthy
• Academically unsuccessful
• Socially inept
• Unhygienic
• Lazy

So a child with a short-term problem may find himself the recipient of all sorts of negative stereotypes, which can be both bewildering and destructive. There is no doubt that children who feel bad about themselves have little self-esteem and therefore care little about what they look like – or have the self-respect necessary to monitor their own health. A 2001 study found that overweight children as young as five can develop a negative self-image, while obese adolescents show declining degrees of self-esteem associated with sadness, loneliness, nervousness and high-risk behaviours. And as I outlined earlier, parents can exacerbate the problem by drawing attention to it, and putting their children on diets. Attempting to control your child's weight by drawing attention to a perceived problem can actually have the opposite result.

But what emotional factors lead to overweight in the first place?

Using food to satisfy emotions

Parents who use food to satisfy their children's emotional needs or to promote good behaviour may, in fact, promote obesity by interfering with their children's ability to regulate their own food intake. Food can take on emotional significance when used to comfort or reward children, and when they are unhappy or suffering the normal ups and downs of growing up they may turn to comfort foods to make themselves feel better. This type of habit is very difficult to shift, and can cause weight to spiral out of control.

If your child wants a food treat when he's down, or appears to be eating more during periods of stress or unhappiness, chances are he's eating for comfort and not to satisfy hunger. Look at your own habits, too. Do you comfort eat or drink? Do you offer your child a sweet or a biscuit to cheer him up? Is a takeaway pizza a reward for doing something well? If children learn to associate food with happiness and good things, they will use it to try to achieve those feelings when they are absent.

Loneliness

Because of changes in family structure and employment over the past couple of decades, children frequently experience disrupted family life and less 'quality time' with their parents. Compared with previous generations, today's youth is more likely to live in divorced or single-parent households, have fewer extended family members (if any) around, have fewer siblings, have an employed mother, spend time in childcare, or spend afternoons home alone. For an ever-growing number of children and adolescents, the 'latchkey' phenomenon adversely affects psychological development, eating style, physical activity and weight status, and may contribute to loneliness. Many kids eat in front of the television – and often do so alone – without any company or interaction with their parents. There is not only no-one on hand to guide meal choices and ensure that a child is eating well, but children are also at the mercy of advertisers, who encourage unhealthy food choices.

THE IMPACT OF PARENTS

According to recent research, parents who tightly control what their children eat might be promoting the exact problems they're trying to prevent – a preference for 'off-limit' foods and a less-than-healthy relationship with food. Researchers found that when exposed to popular snacks like chocolate and ice cream, children whose parents tended to tightly control what they ate were more likely to overeat in the absence of hunger, and express more negative feelings about their eating, than those children whose parents had a more relaxed approach to child feeding.

The findings revealed that in the absence of hunger, nearly all the girls ate snacks, with consumption ranging from 0 to nearly 450 calories. Roughly half reported eating 'too much' and feeling bad about eating at least one or more of the snack foods. Approximately one-third said that they would feel bad if their mother or father found out about what they had eaten.

Other research has also found that highly controlling approaches to child feeding undermine children's ability to develop and exercise self-control over eating. Parental control in child feeding is negatively associated with preschool children's ability to self-regulate their energy intake.

Another study found that when mothers' restrictive control was low, children seem more responsive to internal cues that signal hunger and the feeling of being full following a meal. However, for children whose mothers were restricting their intake, eating was elicited by the presence of 'forbidden' food, even when they were not hungry. This effect was seen most strongly in girls. Mothers whose own eating was 'out of control' used more food restriction with their daughters, and their daughters ate more when not hungry. These findings reveal parallels between the mothers' and daughters' eating style and suggest that restrictive child-feeding practices may effectively transmit an out-of-control eating style from mothers to daughters.

What's your view on your child's diet? And what is your own relationship with food? If you are overzealous about what your child eats your attitude could be part of the problem. Equally, if you are a chronic dieter, pick at your food, refuse to eat certain things or tend to gorge occasionally or use food as treats, you may be sending the wrong message.

Studies have also shown that support from parents and others is a very strong factor in encouraging children to participate in physical activity – so a child who is spending a lot of time alone will not be getting the encouragement to have a healthy lifestyle.

Given that emotional factors affect dietary and physical behaviour, which affects energy balance, it is not surprising that children who suffer from neglect, depression, or other related problems are at substantially increased risk of obesity during childhood and in later life.

Depression

This is a growing problem in children yet, according to some research, depression in children may go unnoticed and untreated. Could your child be depressed? Common signs include children who:
• Lack interest in activities they previously enjoyed
• Criticize themselves
• Are pessimistic or hopeless about the future
• May feel sad or irritable
• May have problems at school that arise from indecision and difficulties with concentration
• Tend to lack energy
• Often have problems sleeping
• May have stomach aches or headaches
• Experience morbid thoughts that may progress to suicidal thinking and even suicide attempts.

As recently as the early 1980s, many psychiatrists believed children were incapable of experiencing depression because they lacked the emotional maturity to feel despondent. In fact most children feel down at times. In the UK, at least two per cent of children under 12 struggle with significant depression – by the teenage years this has risen to five per cent, or one in 20. That equates to at least one depressed child in every classroom. Other studies suggest that, in the course of a year, eight to nine per cent of children between the ages of 10 and 13 suffer from an episode of depression.

For various reasons, some adults find it hard to accept that children may experience unpleasant psychological states such as depression. And the problem is that it does appear to be more common than you might think. A community survey of Australian children found that 3.7 per cent of boys and 2.1 per cent of girls aged six to 12 years had experienced a depressive episode in the previous 12 months.

So what does that have to do with weight? First of all, self-image is enormously affected during an episode of depression, and children, like adults, lose interest in taking care of themselves, or develop a poor body image. Overeating, comfort eating, destructive behaviours and apathy are common characteristics of depression. The problem is, of course, that even short-term depression can lead to a rise in weight that sets kids on course for increased weight gain and the negative feelings that accompany it. The connection between depression and obesity remains unclear, but studies have shown that women with severe mental illness are at increased risk of obesity as well as cardiovascular, endocrine and infectious diseases. Chronic obesity (lasting from childhood into adulthood) is associated with psychiatric disorders such as oppositional defiant disorder (see page 173) and depression. Two major studies indicate that predictors of childhood overweight and adulthood obesity include parental neglect, poverty and childhood stress and depression.

Depression has been aptly described as a 'whole-body illness' because it involves not only changes in mood but in almost every other area of a child's life as well. Depressed youngsters may suffer from problems with sleep, appetite and general health. They frequently complain of vague physical symptoms, such as headaches and stomach aches, for which no medical cause can be found. Depression affects the ability to think, concentrate and remember; as a result, the depressed child's school performance deteriorates and grades begin to drop. Friendships dissolve as depressed children become increasingly withdrawn or, in some cases, irritable and argumentative. The family suffers, too, from the child's moodiness, emotional outbursts and constant whining and complaining.

Depression affects the way a child looks, feels, thinks and behaves. Depressed children often look distinctly unhappy: bright smiles and cheerful grins give way to a glum, mask-like facial appearance. If the predominant mood symptom is irritability, an angry, sullen expression seems permanently fixed on the child's face. Self-

HOW MUCH TIME DO YOU SPEND WITH YOUR CHILDREN?

Research funded by Powergen found that six out of 10 parents do not have time to read to their children before bed. Dr Aric Sigman, the psychologist who ran the study, questioned 84 parents with 150 children to compare reading patterns between generations. While almost three-quarters recalled being read to regularly when they were young, only 40 per cent of their children heard a story most nights of the week. Other researchers have said that a culture of long working hours destroys parents' relationships with their children, making it difficult for them to talk to them or monitor their homework. One common complaint from children is that their parents – especially dads – fall asleep themselves before they have finished reading a story.

Only one in five households enjoys a meal together once a week, and a quarter said they eat together only once a month. The survey of 1,000 households by the Food Foundation, also found that only 15 per cent sat down together every day. A later study by the Consumer Analysis Group, published in April 2001, showed that parents considered this trend to be worrying: more than 80 per cent of parents felt that family dinners were a vital part of home life. Over 33 per cent thought that the dinner table provided the only opportunity to discover what their children were thinking. Despite this belief, only 75 per cent of the sampled group managed a family meal once a week.

Does it really matter if we eat with our kids? Studies show that it does. In particular, a large federal study of American teenagers found a strong association between regular family meals and academic success, psychological adjustment, and lower rates of alcohol use, drug use, early sexual behaviour and suicidal risk.

While most children in the UK claim to take part in regular family-based activities, a fifth of all children reported that they had not done anything with their father in the last week.

In one poll, 21 per cent of teenagers rated 'not having enough time together with parents' as their top concern. Is it any surprise then that today's children feel lonely and seek out comfort in other ways? This must be at least be part of the reason for the trend towards obesity.

CASE HISTORY: # Mark

Mark first put on weight at the age of 11, when he was struggling to make the grade in his exams. His parents insisted that he spend most of his free time studying, and constantly pointed out the importance of his results. He felt stressed and under pressure and, with little exercise to reduce the impact of this, his weight began to steadily increase. He started snacking constantly, even reverting to sneaking food that his parents disapproved of. He ate to reduce the feelings of being out of control and unhappy. He put on more than a stone over three months of inactivity and overeating, and, aware of his growing weight problem, became anxious and depressed – a shadow of the happy, clever child he had once been. He even began to doubt his own ability to achieve good grades. In a nutshell, his self-esteem plummeted as his weight soared.

He finally plucked up the courage to tell his parents that the pressure they had placed upon him was making him unhappy. Not surprisingly, they were very worried and immediately began to reassure him that doing his best was good enough for them.

esteem plummets and the child feels guilty, inadequate and unloved. Loss of energy is common and depressed children often become 'couch potatoes' who do little but watch TV or play video games. A previously agreeable child might become increasingly uncooperative and defiant, refusing to abide by rules at home or in school. When this happens, parents often attribute the difficult behaviour to wilfulness and resort to disciplinary tactics, while the child's underlying problems go undiagnosed and untreated.

In teenagers, symptoms of depression such as moodiness, poor self-esteem and school failure are often chalked up as 'typical teenage behaviour'. If – as is often the case with depressed adolescents – the teenager also falls in with a bad crowd, abuses drugs or alcohol, and runs afoul of family and societal rules, it is even more likely that the real source of the problem will be overlooked. The result? Problems that might otherwise be corrected with treatment may escalate out of control.

Does this sound like your child, either now or in the past? If so, depression may be at the root of your child's weight problem.

Stress

Stress in children is undoubtedly on the increase, even in very young children, such as preschoolers. According to research published in October 2000, children as young as eight describe themselves as 'stressed'. More than 200 interviews conducted by a team from City University in London found unprecedented levels of stress in people of all ages and 'worryingly high' levels in children. More than a quarter of those questioned by the researchers said they were often or always stressed, while half were 'occasionally stressed'. 'We were surprised by the extent of the problem, particularly by the amount of stress reported by very young people,' said Professor Stephen Palmer, who led the study. 'If you had asked eight-year-olds about stress 20 years ago, they would have looked blank. Now they understand the concept and a significant number report experiencing it.' They also found that nearly a quarter of the under-18s interviewed said that they often got stressed, and only one in six never suffered from it.

In 1996, on behalf of the NSPCC, MORI Social Research interviewed a representative quota sample of 998 children aged eight to 15 years old in England and Wales. The aim of the survey was to obtain a contemporary picture of children's experiences of, and attitudes towards, family and social life. Surprisingly, researchers found that stress and anxiety were considered to be normal by almost half of those polled.

When asked about sources and frequency of worries, academic pressures were the most commonplace (44 per cent) for all except the youngest children. Younger children were generally more likely to say they frequently worried about things and a fifth were classified as 'anxious' on a composite scale, compared to one in ten of those aged 12 or over.

There is plenty of research to suggest that our children's emotional health is being seriously affected by stress. So what stresses children? Traditionally, stress has been defined in terms of its cause – in other words, whether it is 'internal' or 'external'. Internal sources of stress include hunger, pain, sensitivity to noise, temperature change and crowding, fatigue and over- or under-stimulation in a child's immediate physical environment. External stressors can include separation from family, change in family structure, exposure to arguing and interpersonal conflict, exposure to violence, experiencing the aggression of others (bullying), loss of important personal property or a pet, exposure to excessive expectations for accomplishment, 'hurrying', and disorganization in a child's daily life events. Although many studies appear to focus on single stressors, such as grief, violence and change, for example, in real life children experience stress from all sorts of directions. And 'multiple stressors' can, of course, have a cumulative effect.

Stress is a strong risk factor for overweight. Children eat to relieve feelings of discomfort and distress, particularly when they don't understand the emotions that they are experiencing or know how to deal with them. In addition, new research suggests that there is a biological link between stress and the drive to eat. Comfort foods – those high in sugar, fat and calories – seem to calm the body's response to chronic stress. In addition, hormones produced when we are under stress encourage the formation of fat cells. Emerging evidence suggests that brain systems that are either affected by stress, or which moderate our response to stress, play a role in disorders of both mood and weight regulation.

Quiz

Is your child stressed?
Answer the questions honestly, placing a tick beside those that apply:
My child:
1 Has unexplained physical symptoms that occur frequently or even constantly, such as headaches, tummy aches, limb or joint pains
2 Suffers from regular constipation or diarrhoea
3 Feels faint, or is subject to fainting
4 Suffers from indigestion
5 Suffers from palpitations
6 Has skin problems

7 Has sweating or clammy hands

8 Seems to pick up every infection going round

9 Takes a long time to reach top form after being ill

10 Always seems tired

11 Finds it difficult to get out of bed in the morning

12 Has mood swings

13 Has a poor appetite

14 Is unusually hungry or obsessive about food

15 Suffers sleep disturbances, such as nightmares, night waking or night terrors

16 Finds it difficult to fall asleep at bedtime

17 Falls asleep during the day

18 Shows a lack of concentration on a regular basis

19 Won't settle down to tasks or focus on short-term projects

20 Is overly sociable and reluctant to spend any time alone

21 Is unsociable, preferring to be alone as often as possible

22 Seems manically energetic at times, and then crashes

23 Seems nervous, fidgety or unable to sit still (not relevant to under-fives!)

24 Is often irritable

25 Becomes angry easily

26 Cries easily

27 Loses patience easily

28 Suffers from temper tantrums (not relevant to under-twos!)

29 Is highly competitive

30 Shirks from any competitive activity

31 Spends free time with 'distractions', such as games consoles, loud music, computers or television

32 Becomes aggressive without warning or explanation

33 Reverts to childlike behaviour, such as thumb-sucking, bedwetting, clinginess

34 Is reluctant to talk about problems

35 Seems anxious, apprehensive or frightened

36 Is often ashamed or embarrassed

37 Suffers from occasional or chronic depression, or generally feeling low

38 Feels helpless and out of control

39 Daydreams more often than usual
40 Becomes obsessive about people, interests or activities
41 Has mentioned suicidal thoughts
42 Worries a lot
43 Is accident-prone
44 Clenches his fist or jaws
45 Grinds his teeth (awake or asleep)
46 Manages time poorly and often panics
47 Withdraws from supportive relationships
48 Is too busy to relax
49 Relies on stimulants, such as colas, sweets, chocolate etc., to keep going
50 Has experienced a dramatic change in weight

If you have ticked more than five of these characteristics, your child is exhibiting symptoms of stress overload. In Chapter 6, I'll look at how you can reduce the stress load and help encourage optimum health and well-being.

Family life

We've already established the fact that families simply are not the supportive, cohesive units that they once were. Parents are busy, extended family members often live hundreds of miles away, children spend increasing amounts of time on their own or in the care of a childminder or nursery, and an increasing number of families are fractured through divorce. These trends have been established across much the same period as the rise in obesity, so it's fair to surmise that children are affected both emotionally and physically by this new way of living. Furthermore, if families are not sitting down to eat together, as is increasingly the norm, there is less regulation of what children eat and little opportunity for parents to set examples and teach valuable lessons. Consider how much time you spend with your child.

TV viewing

The link between television viewing and obesity is now firmly established. One 1999 study found that obesity risk decreased by a whopping 10 per cent for each hour per day of moderate to vigorous physical activity, but increased by 12 per cent for each hour per day of television viewing. This means that every one of those hours that your child spends in front of the TV increases her risk of obesity.

Television viewing is thought to promote weight gain not only because it takes the place of physical activity, but also by increasing energy intake. It encourages unhealthy snacking and a stimulation of appetite at times when your child is not normally hungry – usually because of the amount of food advertising aimed at kids, but also because kids are more likely to eat mindlessly when they are in front of the TV.

Moreover, television viewing during mealtimes is associated with lower levels of fruits and vegetables being eaten (the very foods that are not advertised, of course).

Analysis of the nutritional content of food and drink advertised during children's viewing times demonstrates that over 95 per cent of the products contained high levels of fat and/or sugar and/or salt. The largest categories of advertised food on children's television were confectionery, cakes and biscuits. While fruit and vegetables were not advertised at all, fatty and sugary foods were advertised in proportions up to 11 times higher than the proportion recommended in dietary guidelines. This information is detailed in the report *TV Dinners: What's Being Served Up by the Advertisers* (see Resources page 251). The report illustrates how children viewing Saturday morning TV will see more than twice as many adverts per hour for unhealthy foods as adults viewing after 9pm.

HOW MUCH TV DOES YOUR CHILD WATCH?

The recent publication of the Sustain (the alliance for better food and farming) report, *TV Dinners: What's Being Served Up by the Advertisers*, provides some fairly startling figures. The research compares the nature and extent of television food advertising during children's and adult viewing periods and demonstrates that advertising on children's television presents a grossly imbalanced nutritional message. For this survey, researchers monitored 272 food adverts during nearly 40 hours of commercial TV programming aimed at both children and adults.

It also maintains that the cumulative effect of advertising that portrays unhealthy food and soft drinks as desirable choices, is to reinforce children's bad dietary habits and undermine efforts of parents and health professionals to encourage healthier patterns of eating. Given the current poor state of children's diets, increasing rates of childhood obesity, the high prevalence of dental diseases and scientific evidence that diets high in fats (especially saturated fats), sugar and salt have a detrimental effect on children's current and future health, this selective targeting seems unjustifiable.

But whether it is justifiable or not isn't really the issue here. You may have a great philosophy for health and nutrition in your household, but if your child is watching a great deal of television, chances are that message is being undermined. There is no question that children are affected by advertising and that they feel they need – and then demand – the foods that appeal. This puts parents under great pressure when choosing and preparing family meals, but it also means that when children are given free choice, and their own pocket money, their decisions are unhealthily influenced by advertising. The best way to get round this is, of course, to limit television, but also to sit down with your child and explain how advertising works, how it is designed to make people want to spend money on the things they don't necessarily need, or which may not be good for them, and why the foods that are being advertised are not right for your child or your family. Most kids don't like to think they are being cynically manipulated, so pointing out just what's going on can go some way to getting them on your side. You'll find the website Media Smart (see Resources page 253) an invaluable source of help with this.

No time to play

Studies show that children now play an average of one hour less per day than they did only three years ago. The findings of *America's Children*, a fascinating long-term study published in 2000, reflect the general trend towards children having a more sedentary lifestyle with less opportunity for play. Children are spending more time on average in childcare and school and more time accompanying their parents on errands and in household tasks, hence they have less time for free play. In 1997, children spent about eight hours more per week in childcare, pre-school or school programmes than they did in 1981. They also spent three hours more per week doing household work, including shopping. Children also spent about three hours less per week in unstructured play and outdoor activities than they did in 1981.

On average, children whose mothers worked outside the home tended to spend the most time in school and childcare, and the least time in free play. Altogether, free time – defined as time left over after eating, sleeping, personal care and attending school, pre-school or day care – decreased from 38 per cent to 30 per cent of a child's day. One-quarter of that free time was spent watching television (13 hours per week). Time spent studying increased by almost 50 per cent per week between 1981 and 1997.

The end result is that kids are simply not given free time to explore, relax, run around the garden, meet up with friends and develop active hobbies. Whether parents are concerned about the risk of abduction, traffic or even the threat of paedophiles, they are less likely to allow their children to play away from home unsupervised, and this has resulted in children who become used to staying inside, playing on computers and games consoles, and watching television. The deterioration of inner city neighbourhoods has also led to fewer open spaces, busier streets and more violence, pressuring parents to keep their kids inside – where they are perceived to be 'safe'. They often have to wait for parents to be free to go to the park or meet up with friends, or even to play outside, and given the fact that so many parents have so little time, this type of activity is at a premium. Instead parents are actually encouraging indoor pursuits, which occupy their children without them having to leave the house. The result? Poor levels of fitness and very few active interests, all of which exacerbate weight problems.

And exercise...

Closely related to the trend for less outdoor activity and fewer hours of playtime is the clear reduction in exercise. Kids today simply do not get enough exercise to keep them fit, to keep their metabolisms working well and to burn off the energy from the food they are eating. Exercise is also one of the most effective ways of reducing the effects of stress and of improving mood, and a lack of regular exercise can be part of the reason why our children are experiencing emotional problems that affect their day-to-day lives and their relationship with food.

Of course, it's not just parents who are responsible for the decline in exercise habits. Children are not getting enough exercise through school PE programmes. Primary schools in England and Wales have halved the amount of time allocated to PE in the last eight years. About 33 per cent of boys and 38 per cent of girls aged two to seven are not meeting minimum levels of activity. Furthermore, secondary schools in England and Wales fall behind their European counterparts. Schools in France and Germany, for example, allocate three hours a week to PE classes, while in England and Wales the average secondary school has just two hours of lessons. Officials at Sport England, the government-funded sports council, found that only one in four 5- to 16-year-olds plays any sport regularly.

Despite this, a 1998 study in the UK showed that the majority of children consider themselves 'fairly fit', although less than 25 per cent exercised or were active for more than six hours a week. This indicates that our children are simply not aware of what fitness entails, nor have they been educated about its importance. Furthermore, a recent study found that children walk 80 per cent less than they did just 20 years ago.

Children who do not get enough exercise tend to put on weight on their bellies and chests – in other words, they adopt the unhealthy 'apple shape'. A study looking at fat distribution in 127 normal-weight children between the ages of nine and 17 found that subjects with apple-shaped bodies (fat collected on upper body and stomach) had higher blood pressure and lower levels of 'good' cholesterol than those with 'pear-shaped' bodies (fat collected on hips and thighs). Apart from an unhealthy diet, the major cause of this type of weight distribution was linked to inactivity. Given that evidence of heart disease has been found in three-year-olds, it's fairly clear that patterns are established early in life.

A little exercise can go a long way. One study found that a two-year moderate aerobic exercise programme (involving running 20 minutes per day) for 41 obese boys and girls resulted in a 30–40 per cent decrease in body fat and a 33 per cent increase in lean body mass. That's the type of exercise that kids used to get on a daily basis, but no longer have regular access to, or the inclination to achieve.

Some statistics and facts

The research all points to the same thing: children are getting fatter, and it's making them ill. Let's look at the reality:

• A Gallup poll, conducted on behalf of the BBC, found that almost 40 per cent of the UK population never take any exercise and just as many believe they are overweight or very overweight.

• A study of 1,000 children found that half the girls and a third of the boys didn't even do the equivalent of a 10-minute brisk walk once a week.

• In 1971, 70 per cent of 10-year-old children walked to school. Today that figure is less than 10 per cent.

• Less than half of Britain's children do 30 minutes of exercise a day – the minimum recommended by the government to keep fit and healthy. A survey by Norwich Union Healthcare shows that only one in eight children takes the ideal one hour of exercise a day, although most say they enjoy sport at school.

• One in five does just one to two hours exercise a week and 12 per cent do no exercise outside school.

• Seventy-seven per cent of parents questioned in the same survey thought physical activity was as important as school work and 98 per cent considered it vital for health, but most admitted they never did any sport with their children.

Physical fitness is a vital part of maintaining weight and preventing overweight. If your child is not getting enough exercise, there is no doubt that his weight will be affected.

This chapter has pinpointed some of the main reasons why children are becoming overweight. There are other factors that can play a part, such as eating disorders and conduct disorders, some of which we will touch upon later in this book, as well as societal pressures and expectations that have changed the way we live our lives on a day-to-day basis. However, what is clear from the research is that there are elements of our children's lives and their upbringings that need to be addressed in order for their weight problems to be resolved. Whether your child's problems are largely to do with the type of diet she is eating, too much television and a lack of exercise, or because she is under pressure and suffering from emotional problems associated with growing up, such as peer pressure, exams, or a broken family, addressing the root cause is vital if you are to set your child on the course to good health and a healthy weight.

We've looked at a lot of things that children aren't getting. The next chapter looks now at what they really need. And that starts with a healthy diet.

Chapter Three

The Food Factor

The needs of the average child are straightforward and easily met. However, no-one would argue that bringing up children, and making the correct choices for them, is a simple job. Kids are exhausting, often demanding and normally active beyond the energy resources of many parents. Add to that, too, the fact that as parents we are inundated with information in books, magazines and newspapers, given constant guidance about how to do things 'correctly', and then hit with numerous scare stories in the media which suggest that all of our efforts are in vain, or wrongly directed. Many parents work, juggle family time with jobs and keeping up our homes, plus we are under intense pressure to raise healthy, intelligent, successful and emotionally sophisticated children. It's a tall order and not surprisingly many parents, through exhaustion or confusion, let some things slide.

In an attempt to ensure that our kids are doing their homework, getting a decent education, taking part in stimulating activities and staying out of trouble, we often forget the basics – good nutrition, plenty of exercise and fresh air, good-quality sleep and a strong family relationship. Fresh, home-cooked food is one of the first things to slide in many families – not because of laziness on the part of parents but due to time constraints. Indeed, a multi-million pound business has grown in response to the demand for quick, easy-to-prepare children's food, and the supermarket shelves are lined with products that appeal both to children and busy parents. A godsend, some might think. And even if parents do have a niggling feeling that the sort of food they are feeding their children is not remotely like the diet they had themselves as children – or even particularly nourishing – it's easy to overlook concerns when everyone else's children are eating the same things and your kids seem healthy and well.

Simple needs, like a good night's sleep, also fall by the wayside in our 24/7 society – when parents get home late from work, kids have ludicrous amounts of homework or heavily orchestrated schedules that run well into the evenings. In order for parents to spend some quality time with their children – or even to allow children some free time on their own – bedtimes have slipped and slipped. So too has time for family outings and leisure activities – just the sort of thing that usually involves exercise and fresh air for children. The result is often an erratic lifestyle that undermines the very tenets of family life, and a child's sense of security.

Many of these changes have coincided with the rise in childhood obesity. In the previous chapter we looked at the various factors that can impact on a child's weight, and it's clear that many of them relate to our modern lifestyle and society, our expectations and, to some extent, the decline in family time together.

Kids grow up quickly these days, and make choices about what they eat far earlier than in previous generations. And ironically, the wealth of foods available has led to a generation of fussy eaters, with a limited repertoire of food likes. With advertising influencing their choices, and a new 'louder' voice (the product in some ways of an emphasis on children's rights), children are demanding certain types of foods and getting them.

Today's kids also have clearly defined tastes when it comes to leisure activities, and the advent of technology has meant there is a broad range of non-physical activities to keep them occupied, at the expense of physical exercise. One of the main problems is the fact that many kids are now consumers in their own right, with perceived needs, demands and their own money to spend. While parents haven't exactly lost control, it's a lot harder to persuade a savvy 10-year-old to toe the family line when he is abundantly aware of the options available to him.

So regaining a little control over our children and actively parenting them – guiding them until healthy habits are established and they are genuinely able to make informed decisions on their own – is one of the most important things any parent can do to prevent the factors that lead to obesity from taking hold. It's also the key to taking control of an existing weight problem, because working together as a family is the best and really the only way to make the changes necessary to get your child back on course.

This may all sound like hard work, and lay the responsibility for making changes firmly on the doorstep of busy parents, but the necessary changes are probably more minor than you might expect – and the results are more than rewarding.

The following chapters examine how you can get your kids to eat well, the importance of exercise and a balanced lifestyle, and how you can help them achieve emotional stability. These are the fundamentals of maintaining a healthy weight, preventing a problem before it rears its head, and dealing with weight that has become an issue. Before these topics are covered, it's vital to look at what kids need from a healthy diet.

Good food matters

Our children's diets need to be adjusted not only to balance them in favour of healthier food, to reduce the risk of overweight and get an unhealthy eating pattern under control, but also to ensure that they have the nutrients they need, in the form of vitamins and minerals, to learn, grow, concentrate, and develop physically, emotionally and intellectually. Many parents will grudgingly accept that their children's diets leave something to be desired, and are aware that the food they are serving is often dictated by children's demands, convenience and practicality rather than designed to promote optimum health. Other parents are genuinely surprised to find that the food their children eat may not be as healthy as they think, and that their child's weight problem is a direct result of their diet. After all, other children may appear to eat much the same things and stay slim. What's more, much of the food that is marketed for children very cleverly convinces parents that it is healthy and nutritious. It's important, therefore, to get back to basics.

Breastfeeding

For many parents, it's too late to go back quite this far, but if you are planning to extend your family, it's something to consider very carefully. Studies show that breastfeeding a baby, even if only for a short period of time, may reduce the risk of obesity in later life. A large study from Harvard found that babies fed mainly breast milk were significantly less likely to be overweight by age 14.

Although another study found that breastfeeding had only a minor effect in preventing obesity in children aged three to five (only 16 per cent less likely to be obese), it appeared that breastfeeding did help to prevent later obesity. It's also worth noting that formula-fed babies tend to have faster very early growth and higher insulin concentrations than breastfed babies, which has been related to heart disease in later life. So if you have a choice, breast is a good start in preventing overweight.

Weaning

This might be an event long past for most children, but again you should be aware of recent findings if you're planning to have more children. Recent thinking was that children should be weaned on to solid foods as late as possible, to ensure that they do not develop allergies. However, while this may be beneficial in preventing allergies, a 2004 study found that late weaning can mean that babies become iron-deficient, and suffer deficiencies of other key nutrients. They also tend to be weaned on to unsuitable convenience foods, because they are that much older.

According to Dr Roger Harris, who led the study, poor feeding habits beginning early in life are contributing to the rising levels of obesity. He points to inappropriate weaning of infants and young children's sugar-laden diets as major culprits. Harris says that too many children, especially in inner cities, are at risk of iron deficiency because they don't receive iron-enriched foods as babies and continue as children to subsist on 'convenience' foods that lack the mineral and other nutrients.

Iron deficiency can lead to anaemia, a condition that impairs the blood's oxygen-carrying capacity, causing symptoms such as fatigue. In young children, iron deficiency may also delay the development of language and motor skills. And exhausted, anaemic children are much less likely to be active, which is an important determinant of weight.

For both breast- and bottle-fed infants, experts recommend that parents begin to introduce iron-enriched rice cereals and other foods around the age of five to six months. According to Harris, delaying the introduction of foods, or 'late weaning', often results in iron-poor diets that persist into childhood. 'The end result of late weaning is that babies stay on larger amounts of milk than they need rather than experimenting with food, and so become iron deficient,' he explained. In addition, Harris claims many toddlers and children have high intakes of juice and junk food, which helps promote obesity.

So the best approach is to ensure that your child has an iron-fortified formula, if he is being weaned later than five months, and that sugar-sweetened juices, convenience foods and junk play no role in your child's diet for as long as possible. Certainly no child under the age of two should have anything other than fresh, whole foods.

Irrespective of whether they are fed on formula or solid foods, when children are overfed as babies they lay down fat cells that effectively stay with them for life. Indeed, fat cells cannot be destroyed once they are there, which is one reason why overweight people have so much trouble losing weight and keeping it off. The body stores new fat either by increasing the number of fat cells or by increasing the size of existing cells. It is particularly important to control childhood obesity since new fat cells are primarily formed during childhood. Each year of adding these extra fat cells makes adult obesity more difficult to fight.

Regular meals

The first thing that all children need, regardless of age, are regular meals – breakfast, lunch and dinner, with healthy snacks in between. What you choose to serve at these meals will determine your child's overall health and their weight. So it's important to get it right. Obviously some children are not natural breakfasters, and may sleepily baulk at anything you offer. In the next chapter we'll go through some sample meal plans to help make the process easier, but for now remember that breakfast is a must, even if it's just something small – as long as it's nutritious.

Lunch is often an area of difficulty, too, as many children eat at school and are therefore beyond the control of parents. But there are ways around this. You normally have the option of sending in a packed lunch, the contents of which you can choose with your child to ensure that he likes it enough to eat it. In this way, you can make sure your child is getting a lunch that supplies him with the nutrients he needs and one that is less likely to cause weight problems. Alternatively, you can negotiate with your child to ensure that the choices he makes at school are largely healthy. For example, agree on chips once a week and at least three fruits or vegetables alongside his main course. Many schools will supply you with a menu for the week (and this often stays the same, week in and week out), and you can sit down with your child and work out the best and healthiest options.

Even if a child has a hot lunch at school, it doesn't mean that he can go without a meal for dinner. For one thing, there is a strong possibility that the lunch he chose may have been typical children's fare that did not contain the nutrients he needs. So you'll need to make up for a poor lunch at dinner time. And even if he does eat a good lunch, he'll still need a nutritious dinner. For the record, nutritious doesn't necessarily mean 'hot'. A cold, picnic-style meal can be equally good for your child – and often lower in the types of fats that we want children to avoid. Again, we'll look at some meal ideas in the next chapter.

Snacks are also important for growing children's well-being. They help to sustain blood sugar levels, thus preventing cravings, and help to keep your child's metabolism stable. However, the choice of snacks is crucial – they must not be regarded as 'extras', but as elements of a carefully planned diet. In other words, they must be nutritious, low in unhealthy fats, salt and sugar – and contribute some vitamins and minerals to your child's diet. We tend to think of snacks as being fun foods – crisps, chocolate, biscuits, and so on – so it's not surprising that children are given these treats to get them through the morning at school, or to tide them over when they get home. In the end, they add nothing to a child's diet but empty calories. They also tend to play havoc with blood sugar levels, causing them to soar and then drop, which leads to fatigue, cravings for sweet foods and mood swings (see box opposite).

THE IMPORTANCE OF SNACKS

Most children need snacks to sustain blood sugar and energy levels, and even those who are overweight need them if they are hungry. But – as I've said before – it's the choice of snack that is important. What your child eats between meals is just as important as what he eats for breakfast, lunch and dinner as they all add or detract from his nutritional status and his overall diet. Kids who fill up on burgers, crisps, sweets, chocolates and fizzy drinks between meals will have no room for healthy food, and probably no taste for it either.

Several studies have shown an inverse relationship between habitual frequency of eating (in other words, snacking) and body weight, leading to the suggestion that nibbling may help to prevent obesity. Not surprisingly, this only appears to be the case when the snacks are healthy.

Children can get up to almost one-half of their total energy intake from snacks, and very recent research indicates that providing children with nutritious, low-fat snacks can have a significant impact on their health. In the West, snacking is growing increasingly popular among children, who consume a minimum of up to two snacks per day. However, the most popular snack foods are also the least healthy, such as soft drinks, crisps and chocolate bars. Researchers who led a 2002 study suspect obesity and poor nutrition among US children may be due in part to unhealthy snacking. Simply substituting healthier foods for unhealthy snacks could have a significant impact on children's diets, they claimed.

Skipping meals may seem like a sure way to cut calories and lose weight, but study findings indicate that it may lead to increased snacking on sugary foods, which can pile on the pounds in the long run. A study of young teenagers found that 20 per cent said they ate just two meals a day, mostly lunch and dinner. These meal skippers generally consumed more snacks than their peers did and these snacks were generally high in sugar, fat and salt, and low in fibre.

What's the answer? I may repeat this point often but it is crucial – look upon snacks as a key part of your child's nutritional intake, not as 'treats' or 'occasional' foods. They are likely to form a good part of your child's overall diet, so it is essential that they are healthy. And what compromises a healthy snack? The same things that qualify as a part of a healthy diet: good sources of carbohydrates, proteins and healthy fats. It's a good idea, too, to offer plenty of choice so that your child can satisfy his cravings for a particular type of food, regulate his own food intake and learn to make healthy choices. We'll look at the best snacks for children in the next chapter.

A healthy diet

The best way to illustrate how our diets should be structured is to use a food pyramid diagram, a device first introduced by the US Department of Health and adopted by many other countries. The pyramid opposite is based on the original but includes some specific guidance on the appropriate choice of foods within the various categories. Make a copy of the pyramid and pin it on your refrigerator so that the whole family can see how a good diet should be balanced.

Understanding the pyramid

It's obvious that the foods at the top end are those that should be eaten less frequently, while those further down can be consumed much more freely. Don't get hung up on portions, though. The pyramid acts as a guide to help parents understand which foods should make up the bulk of the diet, and which should be considered to be 'treats' – served irregularly and certainly not on a daily basis.

Since the original food pyramid was put forward, thinking has changed about some categories. Let's look at the latest thinking.

- Fats and oils. While their position in the pyramid suggests that they should be eaten only sparingly – and it's certainly true that too much fat in your child's diet will obviously be laid down as body fat to some extent – the problem is really only with eating too much and the wrong kinds. We now know that some fats, such as olive oil, which is a monounsaturated fat, actually have a positive effect in the body, and their inclusion in your child's diet can actually help to balance the negative effects of less healthy fats. So while it is never a good idea to overload the body with too many saturated fats such as butter, your child does need healthy fats such as olive oil and seed and nut oils. The ones to avoid are trans fats (see page 76).

- Carbohydrates. It was once believed that cutting out fat in favour of carbohydrates would reduce weight and the health problems associated with a high-fat diet. However, this led many people to believe that all carbs are equal. They are not. The carbohydrate servings recommended here are *whole*

SWEETS
and refined
carbs (a very
occasional treat)

FATS AND OILS
olive oil, unhydrogenated
margarines, seed and nut
oils, butter (the type you
choose matters more than
how much your child eats)

PROTEINS
very lean meats, fish, poultry, cheese,
yogurt, nuts, soya products, pulses, seeds
(4–6 servings a day)

FRUIT AND VEGETABLES
(5–9 servings a day; aim for 3–5 servings of vegetables
and at least 4 servings of fruit)

CARBOHYDRATES
should be wholegrain or unrefined (4–9 servings a day)

carbohydrates, not white or refined. So wholemeal breads, wholegrain cereals, brown pasta and brown rice etc., are all included in this category. Cakes, biscuits, white bread and anything that is made with white, refined flour or sweetened, such as some breakfast cereals, pancakes, white pastas and so on should be treated as a 'once in a while' food, rather than part of your child's carbohydrate intake – that's why they're up there at the top of the triangle with the sweets. Obviously a bowl of white pasta with a nutritious sauce is not an evil, but if your child's diet is weighted heavily in favour of white over brown or 'whole', she won't be getting the nutrients she needs, and her blood sugar levels will suffer.

- Fruit and vegetables. The five-a-day message represents an honourable attempt to get people to eat more of these essential foods; however, five should be the absolute minimum to which you should aim. The balance between fruits and vegetables should also be taken into consideration. Vegetables are extremely important and a diet rich in fruit but no vegetables is not recommended (see page 81). Aim for at least three to five servings of vegetables, and at least four servings of fruits.

- Milk, cheese and yogurt. These foods fall into the 'protein' part of the pyramid. It's important to remember that for health reasons, particularly with regard to calcium intake, kids do need between two and three servings of dairy produce every day. That's about half of their protein intake. Many parents make the mistake of cutting out dairy produce altogether, believing it to be too fatty. It's essential and must be included. The remainder of your child's protein intake should come in the form of fish, lean meats, nuts, seeds, beans and other pulses, and eggs.

The components of a healthy diet

Now let's look at the main components of a healthy diet in more detail, so that you can understand which of these foods are best for your child in the fight against weight gain and obesity, and which should be avoided whenever possible. It makes sense to start with fats.

WHAT IS A SERVING?

Don't worry too much about serving sizes. The main thing is to get the balance right. In other words, if your child is eating a variety of different foods, weighted in importance according to the food pyramid, there should be no problem. For guidance, consider the following recommendations.

- From the time an infant starts solids (four to six months of age) until the age of six, the recommended serving size for fruits and vegetables is one tablespoon per each year of their age. So, for example, four tablespoons of sweetcorn would constitute a serving for a four year old. After age six, serving sizes for fruits and veggies are the same as those for adults – about half a mugful. Remember that fruit and vegetable juices also count as servings. For children above the age of two, about 60 ml (2 fl oz) would be an appropriate serving. A few sips is enough for a toddler.

- For other foods, much the same rules apply – the younger the child, the smaller the portions.

- An adult serving of bread would be one slice, $\frac{1}{2}$ a bagel or muffin, 25 g (1 oz) ready-to-eat cereal, $\frac{1}{2}$ mug of porridge, rice or pasta, or 5–6 crackers or oatcakes. A child above the age of six would need roughly the same sized portions. A quarter of a piece of toast would represent a serving for a two-year-old, and so on.

- Protein portions for children above the age of six would be about 50–75 g (2–3 oz), which is about the size of a deck of playing cards. Again, the younger the child, the smaller the portion. If the portion could fit in the hand of the child it's about the right size.

Fats

Despite the impression given by the press, fat is necessary for growing bodies, and a shortage may lead to cravings and health problems. As we discussed in Chapter 2, low-fat products are not of any real benefit in the fight against obesity. Indeed, they teach children that junk food or fatty foods are fine in their diets, as long as their fat content is reduced. For obvious reasons, this does nothing to educate them about healthy eating habits. Low-fat crisps are no better than full-fat crisps, nor are half-fat cheeses a better alternative to the full-fat variety.

Again, it is the type of fat that makes the difference. There are a number of different types of fats and familiarizing yourself with them will help you to make the right choices for your children – and indeed the whole family.

Fats to avoid
Trans fats
The most harmful type of fats are trans fats, the type that most often appear in 'low-fat' or modified foods, as well as most junk and convenience foods – and very often the type aimed at kids. Trans fats are produced through hydrogenation, a chemical process that adds hydrogen to an unsaturated fat, such as a vegetable oil, in order to make it solid or spreadable. Trans fats are strongly associated with an increased risk of heart disease. What's more, they appear to be even worse for health than saturated fats because in addition to raising bad cholesterol, they may lower good cholesterol. They are also now being linked with certain cancers.

Trans fatty acids lengthen the shelf life of products and hence they're commonly found in processed foods, commercial baked goods (such as biscuits, cakes and doughnuts) and many margarines. Of course, foods will not list trans fats in the ingredients list on the label – instead it will say 'hydrogenated' vegetable oil or fat. Some foods are 'partially hydrogenated', which means that they are partially hardened – these too should be avoided because of the high levels of trans fats.

Fats to eat sparingly
Saturated fats
You may be surprised to see this here, as saturated fats have been considered the bad guy for many years – and with some justification. Saturated fats are found in animal products such as butter, cheese, fatty meats, whole milk, cream and ice cream. They are also found in some vegetable oils, such as coconut, palm and palm kernel oils.

A diet high in saturated fat increases the quantity of 'bad' cholesterol in the body and is one of the major risk factors for heart disease. Too much fat also increases the risk of heart disease because its high calorie content increases the likelihood of obesity.

Diets high in fat, especially saturated fat, affect the way your child's body responds to sugar, and increases the risk of type 2 diabetes. Their bodies can cope with a relatively small intake of excess fats, however, if your child gets more than 35 per cent of his calories from fat, he's eating too much. Conversely, any less may not do him any favours either. A 2004 study found that youngsters who ate moderate amounts of any type of fat – 30 to 35 per cent of total calories – weighed less than those who ate either more or less.

Ultimately, a good healthy diet, with some dairy produce (including some butter and cheese), meat, vegetables, poultry, fish, fruits, vegetables and a good source of carbohydrates will never include too much fat. It's the junk food and the convenience foods – which tend to be very high in saturated fats (and trans fats) – that tip the scale and make a diet unhealthy. It's also worth noting that if fats – even saturated fats – are eaten with plenty of fruits and vegetables, their impact is not as dangerous. The reason for this is that fruits and vegetables contain 'antioxidants', which limit the damage that fat has on your child's body. That's just one reason why a balanced diet is so important.

So the occasional ice cream, bit of butter on your child's morning toast or a cheese sandwich is not going to cause problems, even if they do contain saturated fats.

Fats that are OK to eat more often
Polyunsaturated fats
These form the basis of a group of fats known as 'essential fatty acids', and the reason they are called 'essential' is because your child cannot do without them – and neither can you. The problem is that these fatty acids are in short supply in the average Western diet, and in even shorter supply in our children's diets, as they are found mainly in vegetable and fish oils and oily fish. As an essential fatty acid, polyunsaturates have lots of important roles: they help to lower blood cholesterol if they are used in the place of saturated fats, they also help to keep the blood thin, relax blood vessels, lower blood pressure, help maintain the water balance in the body, decrease inflammation and pain, improve nerve function, maintain immunity, affect your child's brain function and metabolism, and balance blood sugar – everything

your child needs to contribute to good short- and long-term health. And in the fight against obesity, some of these roles are crucial. Oily fish, such as salmon, sardines, tuna, mackerel and herring, are good sources. So too are seeds and plant and seed oils. The best are hemp, linseed, safflower, sunflower, corn, pumpkin, walnut, sesame, soya and wheatgerm.

Polyunsaturated oils are healthy unless they are heated, at which point they become unstable and decidedly unhealthy. This is an important consideration. Many people think that using vegetable oils in cooking will add to their children's intake of healthy oils. It won't if it's been heated; in this case it will become a health hazard. Only 'raw' oils are good sources of key nutrients. The best way to increase polyunsaturates is to add lots of oily fish (you can at least try!) and seeds to your child's diet.

Monounsaturated fats

Sources of monounsaturated fats include olive oil, avocados, nuts, seeds and rapeseed oil. Monounsaturated fats are among the healthiest fats, as they are believed not only to lower levels of bad cholesterol, but to boost levels of good cholesterol. They are believed to be one of the main factors in the well-publicized healthiness of the Mediterranean diet, which is linked to increased longevity, reduced risk of cancer and a lower incidence of heart disease and obesity. Incorporate them into your child's diet from an early age – choose olive oil for cooking (it's more stable than a polyunsaturated oil) and offer olives and avocados regularly.

Ground nuts and seeds can be incorporated in your child's diet from the age of about three. It's worth including these elements in a child's diet from a young age, as they can play an important role in maintaining health.

In a nutshell

• The healthiest fats are the naturally occurring non-animal fats that have not been chemically altered. These include polyunsaturated fats (in vegetables oils, fish oils and seeds and seed oils) and monounsaturated fats (found in nuts, olive oil and avocados).

• Saturated fats are OK in small quantities, but are best eaten as natural, largely unprocessed foods (yogurt, milk, butter, cheese and meat) and with fruit and vegetables, which can help to prevent damaging effects. Crisps, baked goods, confectionery, chips and fried foods will contribute too much fat to your child's diet, which is when it becomes unhealthy.

• The unhealthiest fats are any fat or oil from any source that has been hydrogenated, partially hydrogenated, or in any way chemically altered. Avoid these as much as possible.

Luckily, product labelling has made it much easier for us to assess the level of saturated fats in the foods we serve ourselves and our children. That's not to say that we need to read the labels on every single thing we eat. Look at a few products from the supermarket shelves or your cupboard at home to get an idea of the types of products that are high in saturated fats. Fried foods, mayonnaise, pizza, burgers, many baked goods such as cakes and biscuits, and cooked meats such as salami, are all high in saturated fats. These types of processed sources of saturated fat need to be kept to a minimum.

Carbohydrates

Carbohydrates are as wildly different as fats. And, just as good fats are vital to health, so too are good carbs. Unfortunately, bad carbohydrates form a great deal of our 'junk food' intake, and they tend to act as 'anti-nutrients', which means that they undo all the good effects of the healthy foods we eat.

Carbohydrates are energy food and are the body's main source of fuel. There are two main kinds: refined and complex (unrefined). You can guess which are the good carbs and which are the ones we need to avoid.

Good carbohydrates

Complex carbohydrates include:
• Vegetables and fruits
• Wholemeal unrefined flour
• Wholewheat pasta

- Brown rice
- Wholemeal bread
- Wholegrain breakfast cereals
- Porridge oats
- Pulses
- Barley

The message is to eat unrefined carbohydrates. They provide a sustained source of energy, which means that they take longer to digest and assimilate and they contain vitamins and minerals, and proteins as well, making them excellent forms of balanced nutrition. If it's white, it's not likely to do you any good at all.

The carbs to avoid

Refined carbohydrates supply energy, but they are quickly assimilated, causing a sudden energy boost, and a subsequent fall. You've seen the effects of refined carbohydrates after a birthday party – children eat cakes, biscuits and lots of sweets and become manically energetic. A short time later, it all falls apart as their blood sugar levels slump. This crazy rise and fall can cause mood swings, irritability, temper tantrums, lethargy and tears.

After school, children are often tearful and tired. This is caused by low blood sugar. In other words, they are hungry and need more fuel to raise blood sugar levels. Children whose lunches have been based around refined carbohydrates (including white bread, biscuits, sweets, jellies and soft drinks) will have a noticeably worse post-school slump than those children whose lunches included wholemeal breads or pastas, vegetables, fruit and fresh juices. Don't be tempted to offer a quick pick-me-up in the form of a sweet or a chocolate. The symptoms will improve instantly, but you'll have showdown time well before dinner, as the levels slump again.

Quite apart from the blood sugar issue, refined carbohydrates have had the majority of their nutrients stripped from them in the refining process. Almost all chromium, for example, is lost when flour is refined. Why do I mention chromium in particular? It's the mineral that governs our glucose tolerance levels – aka, blood sugar. Other big losses are calcium, B vitamins, iron, zinc and potassium. Manufacturers would have us believe that adding a few token

FRUITS OR VEGETABLES?

It's extremely important that your child gets as many servings of fruits and vegetables per day as possible. Not only are they rich in key nutrients but they also contain fibre, which improves digestion and helps to slow down the transit of sugars in food into your child's bloodstream.

But it's important to remember that fruit cannot take the place of vegetables. Many parents make the mistake of assuming that several servings of fruit will make up for the fact that their child is not eating vegetables. However, there are several reasons why this thinking is not correct. First and foremost, although fruit is very nutritious, it can be relatively high in sugars (meaning that it has a higher GI, or glycaemic index), which can lead to cravings and high blood sugar. It is, therefore, important to choose your child's fruit carefully. Secondly, although it is rich in many vitamins (including loads of vitamin C) and some minerals, fruit is not quite as nutritious as vegetables when considering overall nutrient levels. Vegetables contain many key minerals and trace elements that are necessary to health – in particular the functioning of your child's metabolism and endocrine systems, which can affect weight. They also tend to be much lower in sugars and very high in fibre.

So it's important to get the balance right. Aim for at least one serving of vegetables for every serving of fruit. If you can't manage that, look at the GI of fruits you are serving and try to choose those that are lower in sugar. Pineapple, mango, grapes and banana, for example, tend to be relatively high in sugars (for fruits), whereas strawberries, raspberries, plums, apples, pears, rhubarb, cherries, apricots, peaches and pears tend to be lower. Remember, too, that when fruits are 'juiced', they lose their fibre content, which is one of the elements that slows down the transit of sugars into the bloodstream. Therefore orange juice will have a higher GI than oranges. And dried fruit tends to be very high, as the sugars become concentrated. When you do serve high GI fruits it's a good idea to serve protein – for example, some yogurt or nuts – at the same time (remember, protein also slows down the transit of sugars).

Vegetables have GI ratings as well, and it's important to get a balance between those that are relatively high in sugars and those that are lower. This shouldn't prove too problematic as most vegetables do fall in the low GI category (see page 85). However, those with a higher GI – for example, baked potatoes, cooked carrots and parsnips – are favourites with many kids so avoid serving them day in day out.

vitamins and minerals to children's breakfast cereals, breads and even biscuits balances the refining process. It doesn't. Adding two or three nutrients to a food that has been stripped of at least 15 does not make it a healthy alternative. Furthermore, these nutrients are not absorbed and assimilated as easily as they are when eaten as a natural part of a food, so many are simply lost in your child's urine. Refined carbohydrates include:

- White sugar (and everything that contains it, including sweets, fizzy drinks, squashes, jams and jellies, cakes, biscuits, chocolate, breakfast bars, breakfast cereals, pies, tarts and most baked goods – the majority of some children's diets)
- White flour (and everything that contains it, including bread, pasta, breakfast cereals, crackers, biscuits, cakes and pies)
- White rice

So you can see why the average child's diet is causing problems. The majority of it is not only based on too many saturated fats, but also on refined carbohydrates, which make kids fat. We explained the main reason for this in Chapter 2 – too much energy floating around affects blood sugar, and is laid down as fat. So even if the carbohydrate products you eat read 'low-fat', they can still make you and your kids fat.

Sugar

Sugar is pretty much pure, refined carbohydrate, which means that it is something that we need to exclude from our children's diets. Sugar has been viewed as an evil for quite some time now. Not surprisingly manufacturers have got smart and started calling sugar by its various generic names, including sucrose, glucose, fructose, lactose, galactose and others in an attempt to ease the blow.

But why is sugar so bad?

- First, sugar has a strong depressive effect on the immune system. According to a 1997 study, as little as six teaspoons a day can reduce the immune response by 25 per cent. Most common foods – particularly those geared towards children – contain a substantial amount of sugar, which can have a dramatic effect on our children's health.

- As we've already seen, sugar causes blood sugar to rise dramatically, which results in the 'hyperactive' symptoms witnessed following a birthday party or even just a packet of sweets. Following the rise, there is a dramatic slump, which causes the other set of familiar symptoms – tearfulness, fatigue, temper tantrums and lack of concentration. This rise and fall can play havoc in any household, and it is simply not good for children to be at the mercy of these types of mood swings.

- Sugars provide calories and no other nutrients, and they damage the enamel of the teeth, causing decay.

- Foods high in sugars are also often high in saturated fats (biscuits, chocolate bars, cakes, pastries, for example), which can lead to overweight, heart disease and even diabetes.

- One of the reasons why sugar leads to overweight is the fact that excess quantities are laid down as fat. A high-sugar diet has been linked with obesity, cardiovascular disease and type 2 diabetes.

- Most importantly, however, the extra calories of sugars often displace more nourishing food in the diet. Diets high in sugar are also often high in fat and low in fibre. If your children fill up on sugary foods, they are likely to be at risk of vitamin and mineral deficiencies, and these can cause imbalances that lead to weight problems.

What should you do?

Remember that kids get far more sugar than they need in even the most healthy diet. Sugar is found in almost everything from ketchup, tinned sweetcorn, soups and pasta sauces, fresh fruit and breads, to cereals (even some of the healthiest, wholegrain brands), many yogurts and almost all convenience foods. And that's without even mentioning the obvious sources, such as squash, jam, jelly, sweets, chocolate, cakes, biscuits and other treats. In many cases, even crisps contain some sugar!

Begin by cutting out the obvious sources. Don't, for example, be tempted to sweeten cereal with sugar. If sugar falls within the first three or four ingredients on a particular food's label, you can be certain that it contains too much for children. Some foods are surprisingly high in sugar. Even so-called healthy breakfast bars can have many different types of sugars, as can cereals and fruit juice drinks.

If sugar is on the label of a food that doesn't need it, such as a processed meat, a tinned fruit or vegetables, or even juice, don't buy it. Obviously some treats, such as chocolate biscuits, have to contain some sugar, but look for a brand with a reduced sugar content (though not one that contains an artificial sugar substitute instead). Many manufacturers have made an effort to cut out sugar, so seek these out as your first choice.

The GI link

In the last chapter we looked at the fact that foods with a higher glycaemic index (GI) had a greater impact on blood sugar (by raising it) than those with a lower GI. And this is important, because high GI foods not only stimulate hunger and cause overeating, but they lead to an increase in blood sugar that can then only be laid down as fat. They also affect the way our children's bodies deal with sugar in general. It is for this reason a high GI diet has been linked with obesity, cardiovascular disease and type 2 diabetes. And not even a gram of fat in sight!

So how do you work out the GI content of food? It's beyond the scope of this book to list the GI rating of every food, but let's look at ratings for some popular foods, so that you get the idea.

The speed at which a food releases its sugar into the bloodstream is given a value from 1 to 100 – 100 being the fastest (pure glucose has a GI value of 100) and 0 the slowest. The higher a food's number, the faster it releases sugar into the bloodstream and the bigger the impact on blood sugar and, in the long run, weight. You'll notice from the list opposite that there are plenty of healthy foods with medium GI indexes – and a few in the high category. The secret is to choose as many lower GI foods as possible and keep the higher ones to a minimum. And there's also another way to balance it. It seems that eating protein (such as nuts, seeds, lean meats, cheese,

THE GIs OF COMMONLY EATEN CARBS

High GI		Low GI	
Glucose	100	Popcorn	55
French bread	95	Brown rice	55
Lucozade	95	Spaghetti	55
Baked potato	85	Sweetcorn	55
Cornflakes	83	Mangoes	55
Rice Krispies	82	Sweet potato	54
Pretzels	81	Banana	54
Rice cakes	77	Kiwi fruit	53
Cocopops	77	Orange juice	52
Doughnuts	76	Porridge	49
Chips	75	Baked beans	48
Corn chips	74	Peas	48
Mashed potato	73	Instant noodles	47
Puffed rice cereal	73	Grapes	46
White rice (boiled)	72	Oranges	44
Bagel (white)	72	All bran	42
Sultana Bran	71	Apple juice	41
White bread	71	Plums	39
Medium GI		Apples	38
Shredded Wheat	69	Wholemeal spaghetti	37
Wholemeal bread	69	Pears	37
Croissant	67	Whole milk	34
Pineapple	66	Chickpeas	33
Cantaloupe melon	65	Yogurt	33
High-fibre crispbread	65	Dried apricots	31
Couscous	65	Soya milk	30
Bread (rye)	64	Kidney beans	29
Muesli bar	61	Lentils	29
Ice cream	61	Fructose	23
Pizza (cheese)	60	Cherries	22
Honey	58	Cashews	22
White pita bread	57	Peanuts	14
New potatoes	57	Lettuce	10
Muesli	56	Mushrooms	10

dairy produce, or eggs, for example) at the same time as you eat higher GI foods slows down the rate that the sugars are released into the blood. So, in other words, protein can effectively lower the GI rating of a food. Sound complicated? It's not. If your child has a white bread sandwich with jam, his blood sugar will soar – the reason is that jam and white bread both have very high GI ratings. But if you give your child a white bread sandwich with chicken and salad, or even cheese, you can slow down the rate at which the sugar in the white bread hits your child's bloodstream.

Generally, a GI of 70 or more is considered high, a GI of 56–69 is considered medium and a GI of 55 or less is thought of as low. Don't worry about sticking solely to the low GI foods at all times. Be aware of which foods are likely to cause blood sugar to rise and potentially lead to weight problems and ensure your child is not overeating these. And if blood sugar or an overabundance of carbohydrates is likely to be at the root of your child's weight problem, you can now make some small adjustments to ensure that that lower GI foods form the basis of most snacks and meals and any high GI foods are accompanied by good-quality protein.

Salt

Children are getting far more salt than they need in their daily diets. For example, bread contains a whopping 500 mg per slice, cornflakes contain more than 900 mg per bowl and even Cheddar cheese comes in at a 335 mg per 50 g (2 oz). The main offenders are processed foods, such as crisps and other snacks, and ready-prepared meals.

The UK government's Scientific Advisory Committee on Nutrition recommends that daily salt intakes do not exceed the following:

• Baby aged up to six months old less than 1 g per day

• Baby aged 7–12 months 1 g per day

• Child aged 1–6 years 2 g per day

• Child aged 7–14 years 5 g per day

• Adult (aged 14+ years) a maximum of 6 g per day

Too much salt puts a strain on the kidneys and can increase the rate at which calcium is excreted from the body (putting children, particularly girls, at risk of osteoporosis later in life). It has also been linked with high blood pressure, strokes, heart disease and stomach cancer. Unfortunately, kids tend to develop a taste for salt and this increases their cravings for junk foods and other processed meals.

Even supermarkets have begun to take note. Sainsbury's in the UK, for example, has just pledged to reduce the salt content of their salt and vinegar crisps, while Asda is also taking steps to reduce the salt content of a variety of its products. At present, bread contributes up to 25 per cent of an adult's average daily intake – and almost 50 per cent of that of children. As a result, supermarkets are now offering bread with a substantially reduced salt content. Look for these brands next time you're at the supermarket.

Many foods, such as breakfast cereals, are surprisingly high in salt – so check those food labels. Once you cotton on to the problem foods, you can exclude them or limit them in your child's diet.

Protein

Proteins are made up of different combinations of 22 separate amino acids, which our bodies need to function and, of course, to carry on living! A lack of protein in the diet retards growth in children and causes a decrease in energy. So if your child is lethargic, a lack of protein may be part of the problem. However, there doesn't seem to be a real problem with the *amount* of protein most children get in our society. But their diets have shifted in favour of carbohydrates (in the form of pizza, pasta, instant noodles, potato chips, sandwiches and so on) and the protein they do get is often coated in breadcrumbs (chicken nuggets or goujons) or served in a bun and is not good quality.

By good-quality protein, I mean fresh fish, poultry, meats, eggs, cheese, yogurt and so on, rather than the processed, ready-prepared stuff. It's also important to include some sources of vegetable proteins, such as beans, nuts, seeds and pulses (most kids love chickpeas, for example).

Ideally, kids should have protein in all three main meals. A half a chicken breast is an ideal serving size for a child under eight, while a whole one would be about right for kids older than that. A serving tends to be something that fits roughly in the palm of the hand of the person eating it, so you can also choose to gauge it that way.

FOOD ADDITIVES

Parents are right to be concerned about the additives and preservatives in foods. Not only are they now known to affect mood, energy levels and health on all levels, but they can also affect your child's weight. The first reason is that they can leave a child feeling moody and out of sorts – so they're unlikely to be cooperative and want to engage in healthy activities. What's more, the additives in our foods are chemicals, not nutrients, and are therefore neither utilized nor eliminated by the body. They are stored in the body, and can upset the fine balance of your child's body chemistry – which includes their blood sugar levels and metabolism. Natural foods do not contain artificial additives; processed and junk foods do. If your child eats too many of the latter, in any form, his health will suffer. Let's look at why.

12 KEY 'ADDITIVES' TO AVOID AND THE HEALTH RISKS RELATED TO THEM

1. Hydrogenated fats – cardiovascular disease and obesity
2. Artificial food colours – allergies, asthma and hyperactivity; possible carcinogen
3. Nitrites and nitrates – these substances can develop into nitrosamines in the body, which can be carcinogenic (cancer-causing)
4. Sulphites (sulphur dioxide, metabisulphites and others) – allergic and asthmatic reactions
5. Sugar and sweeteners – obesity, dental cavities, diabetes and hypoglycaemia, increased triglycerides (blood fats) or overgrowth of Candida albicans (a yeast-like fungus)
6. Artificial sweeteners (Aspartame, Acesulfame K and Saccharin) – behavioural problems, hyperactivity and allergies; possibly carcinogenic. The government

Add to that two or three handfuls of vegetable sources of protein every day and you can be sure that your child is getting a good balance of different proteins, which will give him the nutrients he needs.

Healthy drinks

This is a source of confusion for many parents – the number of soft drinks, juice drinks, juice concentrates and even flavoured waters on the market make it difficult to know what is healthy and what is not.

Let's get one thing straight, fizzy drinks are not healthy. They are largely made up of chemicals and sugars that can not only cause overweight, but a host of other problems, including tooth decay cautions against the use of any artificial sweetener by children and pregnant women. Anyone with PKU (phenylketonuria – a problem with metabolizing the amino acid phenylalanine) should not use aspartame (Nutrasweet).

7. MSG (monosodium glutamate) – common allergic and behavioural reactions, including headaches, dizziness, chest pains, depression and mood swings; also a possible neurotoxin (neurotoxins interfere with the proper functioning of the nerves)
8. Preservatives (BHA, BHT, EDTA, etc.) – allergic reactions, hyperactivity, possibly cancer-causing; BHT may be toxic to the nervous system and the liver
9. Artificial flavours – allergic or behavioural reactions
10. Refined flour (excessive) – carbohydrate imbalances, altered insulin production
11. Salt (excessive) – fluid retention and increased blood pressure
12. Olestra (an artificial fat) – diarrhoea and digestive disturbances

It's fairly clear that a well-balanced, healthy diet for growing children should contain none of these foods. In small quantities, they are unlikely to do any lasting damage, but given the amount of junk and convenience foods our children eat, the overall impact on their bodies can be significant. One of the keys to addressing a weight problem is to ensure that your child is balanced – both physically and emotionally. As many additives have a negative effect on one or both, their bodies and behaviour will undoubtedly be affected. Including them in your child's diet will only make your efforts to encourage a healthy weight less effective. Where are these foods found? Yes, you've guessed it – in most children's food and almost all junk and convenience foods. So check those labels.

and bone loss, which is very serious in children. As we know from the previous chapter, kids are drinking far too many of these drinks, at the expense of healthier alternatives – and even food. Drinks can be very filling, so it's essential that your children's choice of beverages actually add to their overall nutrition rather than take the place of something more nutritious.

Some fizzy waters have fruit juice concentrates added to them, and these are OK in moderation, but most also have sugars and other chemicals added, which means that they can fill up a child with too many calories that, in the long run, will cause weight gain. If your child must have a fizzy drink, mix plain fizzy water with fruit

CASE HISTORY: Flora

Flora knew she had a weight problem and turned to her mum for advice. What she really wanted was to lose weight without her friends noticing that she was on a diet. Her mother took the opportunity to explain to Flora about various aspects of nutrition and, as a family, they made a concerted effort to change their eating habits. She also explained to Flora that a diet wasn't necessary at all. Although there were a few slip-ups in the first few weeks, and Flora had difficulty giving up salty snacks and chips, especially at school, she did start to feel better. She noticed that she felt less tired and moody, and she had a lot more energy. She also lost a little bit of weight – nothing hugely significant, but over the months, as she continued to grow, her weight stayed the same and she started to slim down.

The best thing was that her friends didn't even notice that she was eating any differently – she still ate lots of food, she just made different choices. And she could justify her choices by explaining that she felt tired when she drank too many fizzy drinks, and that fat irritated her stomach when she ate too much. When they were out after school at the local fast-food restaurant, Flora learned to choose grilled chicken sandwiches without mayo, instead of burgers and chips, and to have a nutritious snack instead of supper because she had, effectively, already consumed a meal.

juice. If they insist on something fizzy, it's the healthiest option.

Squashes are basically water flavoured with sugar syrups. A few drops in a glass of water will help to make it more palatable for picky kids, but chances are your child is having a good few tablespoons, which adds a huge quantity of unnecessary sugar. And not all squashes are equal. Some contain almost no fruit juice at all. If you must use squash, use only a few drops and choose brands with at least 50 per cent (and preferably higher) fruit content. At least your child will be getting some nutrition alongside the wallop of sugar.

Don't forget, too, to take into consideration the sugar in drinks when calculating how much your child is getting in a day. You might be surprised. However, don't be fooled into thinking that going for 'low-sugar' brands is a better option. These simply contain artificial sweeteners in the place of sugars, and that means more chemicals that can interfere with your child's digestion, metabolism and other body processes.

Many children do not eat fruit so fruit juice is an important addition to the diet. In fact, a glass of fruit juice is considered to be a serving of fruit, so it's worth including a fresh fruit juice in your child's diet. This does not mean a fruit 'drink', which is something different altogether. A fruit drink is not pure fruit juice, and it will have other things, particularly sugar or a sugar substitute, added. Concentrated fruit juices (those made from concentrate) seem to be as good as fresh in terms of nutrition. The drawback to fruit juices is that they can be very hard on teeth and, because there is no fibre to slow down the absorption of the natural sugars they contain, some release their sugars into the bloodstream relatively quickly. Therefore dilute them if possible, or serve them only with meals. Food also helps to slow down the impact of the fruit sugars in your child's bloodstream (see also Fruit or Vegetables? page 81).

The best drink of all is water, and water consumption should be encouraged as much as possible. The British Dietetic Association's Paediatric Group advises that the fluid needs of children vary from day to day depending on the weather, how active the children are and what food they are eating. It suggests that children drink regularly throughout the day, having drinks offered to them with each meal and between meals (this amounts to about 6–8 glasses of fluid per day, small glasses for small children and larger for older children). Water has no calories, plus a well-hydrated (well watered!) child is much more likely to perform better. You may also see changes in your child's approach to food. Kids complaining of hunger are often just thirsty. Offer a big glass of cold water and see what happens! It's also worth noting that dehydration makes kids tired, headachy, moody and lethargic – so they won't be bursting with the energy necessary to sustain a good, active lifestyle. (See page 117 Encouraging Children to Drink Water.)

The National Diet and Nutrition Survey of young people in 2000 found that four out of 10 primary-aged children did not drink any plain water during the course of one week. The consumption of soft drinks by four- to six-year-olds was found to be 10 times higher than plain water consumption and children aged seven to 10 drank about seven times as many soft drinks as plain water. Four- to six-year-olds consumed three times more soft drinks than milk. Again, this increase in soft drink consumption coincides with the relentless rise in obesity. Making a small change in what your child drinks – from sweetened drinks to water – can cut their sugar load substantially, their calorie load by up to half, and have a dramatic impact on their overall health and temperament.

Milk is nourishing and thirst-quenching. Some experts recommend that you switch to half-fat or semi-skimmed milk after the age of two, to keep levels of fat down. This is particularly important if your child drinks a lot of milk. Interestingly, one study found that milk, which is a low GI beverage, seems to protect overweight young adults from becoming obese. It appeared that despite the calories, youngsters who have dairy food regularly seem to have a lower risk of becoming overweight. Lynn Moore, an epidemiologist at Boston University School of Medicine, found that eating just two servings of dairy food a day is linked to a substantial reduction in adolescent fatness. Childhood dairy intake has been failing for the last 20 years, in part as youngsters' preferences have switched from milk to sugary soft drinks. During this time, soft drink consumption has risen by a whopping 300 per cent.

Another factor, though, has been fat phobia. Youngsters 'consume less and less as they get older', says Moore. 'Adolescent girls in particular are concerned about eating dairy because they think it will make them fat.' However, her research found that just the opposite is true. Several studies – including Moore's – have also shown that children and adults who consume adequate amounts of dairy foods have lower blood pressure. Some researchers have put adults on diets with increased dairy produce and found, to their surprise, that they also seem to lose weight. Just how dairy produce might moderate weight gain is a mystery. Moore speculates that calcium or some other nutrient in milk might help influence the way the body stores energy in fat cells. Or perhaps dairy foods simply make children feel less hungry. So don't be tempted to remove milk or dairy produce from your child's diet in an attempt to encourage weight loss. It may have the opposite effect.

How's your cooking?

The way you cook your children's food can make a big difference to the amount of fat it adds to their diet.

Frying is pretty much a no-no – not only because it adds extra calories in the form of oils used, but also because heating oils oxidizes the fats and turns them into trans fats (see page 76). It also destroys almost all the nutrients. If you must fry foods, stir-fry using only a little olive oil and never heat it to smoking point. A stir-fry with a little olive oil and a few tablespoons of water can be a great way to cook foods quickly so that they maintain their nutritional value – and absorb less oil. Deep-frying is worst of all, particularly if you are trying to monitor your child's weight.

Grilling, baking and roasting foods is an excellent way of cooking them, as these methods rarely require extra fat. Most children won't know the difference! If you are serving chips, for example, oven chips (home-prepared if possible – see page 109) have less than a third of the amount of fat of those that are deep-fried or even shallow-fried. Grilling rather than frying a chicken breast also means a reduction of up to half the calories.

Microwaving food obviously doesn't add any unnecessary fat, and can be a quick way of cooking vegetables; however, it does destroy a huge percentage of the nutrients – and at least part of the reason for changing the way you and your child eat is to do with nutrition rather than just controlling weight. Similarly, boiling can quickly cook foods without the need for extra fat, but the quality of the cooked food will be poor. Just 5 minutes of boiling reduces the thiamine (a B vitamin) content of peas by up to 40 per cent. Similarly, boiling cabbage reduces its vitamin C content by up to 75 per cent. Steaming food with just a little water is your best bet, as it not only retains the most nutrients, but also requires no fat.

It's also a good idea to offer at least some of your child's fruit and vegetable servings raw. These are a great source of fibre, which fill children up and improve digestion, and raw foods are also much more nutritious than cooked.

Try to cut down on fat wherever possible when cooking, and leave out the salt, too. Use herbs, spices, pepper, fruit juice, lemon juice and even tasty vinegars to flavour food – marinate meat before cooking to make it more palatable and easier for children to chew, and season other foods while cooking to give them flavour.

Cooking sauces don't need to be fattening, either. Stir in some fresh yogurt or crème fraiche with a little stock or even wine (cooking burns off the alcohol, which makes it safe for children over the age of five), or use fresh tomatoes or tomato purée in the place of sugary pasta sauces. Chopped herbs or spices will add all the flavour you need. It's also a good idea for kids to get used to the taste of fresh foods – many children's palates have become accustomed to the salty, over-processed taste of convenience and junk foods, and it can take some time for them to get used to the consistency and flavour of fresh foods. If you have to, allow liberal use of condiments such as ketchup, chilli sauce or even sweet and sour sauce (although try to find relatively low-salt varieties) to get them used to your home-cooked, fresh foods, and then gradually cut these down too.

How does your child's diet add up?

Many of us believe we are eating well until we stop and look at our diets in detail. The same goes for our children. If they are older they may well be eating at school, or out with friends. Younger children and babies may be fed by a childminder or at a nursery, and we may not be aware of exactly what they are getting.

The best place to start is to analyse your child's diet for a week. Write down everything they eat in as much detail as you can. You might have to rely on their memory to some extent, or on the willingness of a nursery or minder to supply details, but it's important that you come up with as accurate a picture as possible.

For each day, score your child's diet according to the following criteria:

• For every serving of fresh fruit and vegetables (and their juices), give them 2 points

• Add an extra point for any servings that were raw

• For every serving of wholemeal bread, wholewheat pasta, brown rice, oats, barley, rye, corn, pulses, unsweetened breakfast cereal or potatoes, add 2 points

- For every serving of good quality protein – fish, lean meat, chicken, turkey, cheese, milk, yogurt, tofu, nuts, nut butters (sugar free), seeds or pulses – add 2 points

- For every full glass of fresh water, add 1 point

- No points should awarded for any servings of white bread, pasta or rice

- For every serving of food that was processed (for example, processed meats and cheeses, shop-bought baked goods, including biscuits), subtract 2 points

- For every serving of food that was fried (including chips), or purchased 'ready to serve', subtract 2 points

- For every serving of crisps, potato or maize snacks, chocolate-coated or sweetened cereals, chocolate, sweets and non-dairy ice cream, subtract 2 points

- For every serving of jam, jelly, packet and tinned soups, subtract 2 points

- For every serving of fizzy drinks, artificial fruit drinks and squashes, subtract 2 points

Interpreting the result

Work out your child's total.

A score of over 40 indicates a brilliant diet – lots of balance and plenty of the most important foods.

A score of 30–40 suggests your child has a fairly good diet, but look at ways to improve it even further.

A score of 20–30 indicates that your child's diet needs improving. Your child will be missing key nutrients. Look at the foods that offer the most points (the fruits, vegetables, proteins and unrefined carbohydrates). By bumping up those, you can balance an otherwise unhealthy diet.

A score of 10–20 is very poor. Major changes need to be made to ensure that your child is getting the nutrients she needs to grow and develop.

Less than 10 equals desperately unhealthy. Your child's health will be seriously affected unless you take steps to redress the imbalance.

This is much the same idea as keeping a food diary. Unless you know what your child is eating, you'll never be able to recognize unhealthy patterns and make the necessary changes. It's worth repeating this exercise every week or so for the first couple of months, to keep tabs on your child's diet. Older children can help by doing this themselves (as long as they agree to be honest!) – and you can take part too. You may be surprised to find that your own diet isn't as good as you thought.

Does this all sound impossible to manage on a tight schedule, and with faddy eaters in the house? It isn't as hard as you'd think. In the next chapter I'll look at how to teach children to eat well – how to put all of this information together to ensure that your child gets the nutrients he needs to grow, learn and, most important of all, maintain a healthy weight.

Chapter Four

Teaching Kids to Eat Well

I f every parent had the time to prepare home-cooked, fresh meals on a daily basis, and was able to keep a 24-hour watch on what their children were eating and undertaking in their spare time, then obesity would simply not be the problem that it is today. Many parents have let things slide; not because they don't care, but because they simply didn't realize the importance of getting a child's diet right – nor do they always have the time in which to do so.

So we'll start from the premise that you are busy. You may have faddy eaters in the house, a child who has adopted an unhealthy attitude towards food or one who is addicted to snacks and junk food. You may have an ad-hoc food policy in your household, where everyone eats pretty much what they want when they want, fitted around the busy schedules of all family members. Your kids may also have little understanding of what unhealthy foods do to their bodies or, indeed, what constitutes an unhealthy food.

Our parents undoubtedly had it easier. Many of us grew up in households where at least one parent, usually the mother, was at home to prepare a meal three times a day. Convenience and junk foods existed, but on a much smaller scale, so there weren't the same temptations to resort to them in the place of healthy fare. We usually ate together as a family and, being more active, were generally hungry enough to eat what was put in front of us.

Today, it's a whole different ballgame, with a new set of rules for kids and parents alike. So how does the average parent create and maintain a healthy diet in the face of the pressures of time, advertising, kid power, peer pressure and the wealth of unhealthy food on the market? It is possible, but it does take a little extra work on your part, and that of your whole family – not a ridiculous amount of work, but at least some effort. If you are reading this book, you are already concerned enough about your child to do something to help him with his weight. And concern and interest are enough to get you started.

In this chapter we'll look at how to put together the basics of nutrition to devise a healthy eating plan that will work for the whole family, and how to teach basic nutrition to children so that they understand the impact of what they are eating and learn to make the correct choices. We'll work on those faddy eaters, to change eating habits that may be affecting their weight, and we'll examine how to create a healthy 'food environment' in your home, so that your children develop a good relationship with food. Let's start by looking at your kitchen cupboards.

Stocking up

There are no two ways about it – if you buy junk food, convenience foods or unhealthy snacks, your kids are going to eat them. You cannot develop a healthy eating plan with cupboards full of rubbish. It won't work. The temptation will be too great for children to resist, and you may also be tempted to give in to their demands even if there are other options available. If a child wails, begs and argues for chips or chicken nuggets for long enough, chances are that most parents will give in eventually. But the reality is that if you don't have these foods in your house, you can't.

All the time I hear stories of parents who are bewildered by the fact that their children will only eat 'chocolate spread sandwiches', 'chips', 'chocolate cereals' or 'spaghetti hoops'. Huh? If you don't buy these foods, they simply can't eat them. It's time to face up to the fact that parents do have the ultimate control over what their children eat in the house, and it is our responsibility to ensure that our children eat well. It's not gluttony that makes a child fat in most cases, but a poor diet. And that is something that you do have the power to change under your own roof.

So clear out those cupboards and the cook-chill drawers of your freezer. If you don't feel comfortable throwing out perfectly good food, then run your stocks down as you begin to incorporate a new eating programme. And then don't be tempted to replace such foods. Many of us make the mistake of hitting the same aisles in the supermarket week on week, like robots, buying exactly the same foods – mega packets of crisps, sweets, chocolate spread, cakes, biscuits, tinned spaghetti, frozen chips and pizzas, ready-prepared burgers, sweetened cereals, fizzy drinks, high-sugar fruit squashes and lots of other unsuitable junk.

So what should you buy?

Based on what we learned in the previous chapters, it's clear that junk foods have no place in our children's diets. Start with fresh foods – lean meats, fish, lots and lots of fresh fruits and fresh or frozen vegetables, some pulses (such as chickpeas or baked beans), wholemeal bread, cheese, unsweetened cereals, butter, milk, pure fruit juice, eggs, pasta (preferably wholewheat), rice (preferably brown), rice cakes (again preferably brown), yogurt, dried fruit, nuts and seeds. If you are weaning children off an unhealthy diet, you may want to buy a small packet of biscuits or crisps and a few snack-sized bars of chocolate – a bag of oven chips is OK, too. If you have a busy lifestyle and have to resort from time to time to convenience foods, look for good-quality brands with a low salt and saturated fat content. And avoid anything with the word 'hydrogenated' on it, as this will contain the most unhealthy fats – trans fats.

Avoid shopping with your children at this stage if you can, as they will undoubtedly persuade you to add other goodies to your trolley, or beg for old favourites. You need a clean slate to do this properly, and that means filling up the house with the type of food you actually want your children to eat.

Many parents will now be baulking at the idea of preparing a freshly cooked meal three times a day. Time is often at a premium, and coming home after a busy day of work to a household of starving kids and then taking an hour to prepare something nutritious may be impossible. There is no doubt that it's easier just to stick a pizza in the oven and call it a day. But it's time now to face up to the fact that this type of approach to food teaches our children nothing about nutrition, and fills them with the types of foods that will either make them fat – or have made them fat already.

It needn't be time-consuming or expensive to prepare and eat fresh foods. In fact, the cost of convenience and junk foods can be exorbitant. If you stick to the basics, you'll find that your shopping bill actually goes down. If you have a freezer it makes sense to buy special offers when possible, and to make extra quantities of healthy foods for standby meals when you are too busy to cook. And as for time, it's a fallacy to believe that healthy food has to be cordon bleu with an hour of preparation time. Grilling a chicken breast, baking a potato and putting together a salad takes very little time. On the following pages you'll find lots of ideas for healthy meals that will help to keep your family's weight on target, and none of them takes an enormous effort to prepare.

Before we get onto the nitty-gritty of actual meals here are a few premises to remember:

- Stick to the food pyramid (see page 73) when considering your child's overall daily intake.

- Start with vegetables and fruit – if your child is getting over five servings a day, and preferably more, she'll be filled up with good, nutritious basic foods that will leave her less hungry.

- Try to incorporate at least two or three fruits and/or vegetables at every meal and be careful that you provide a balance; remember – don't neglect the vegetables in favour of fruit.

- Next choose a good source of protein – some chicken, fish, beans or lean meats, such as trimmed pork chops, lamb chops or even lean mince.

- Try to choose unrefined carbs – brown rice, wholewheat pasta, wholemeal bread, potatoes etc.

- Go for water, juice or milk for meals – if water is not popular in your house (and that is something that can be addressed; see page 117), then add a few *drops* of high-fruit squash or pure fruit juice for flavour or a squeeze of fresh lime or lemon juice.

- Dessert or pudding does not have to be off the menu – yogurt, fruit, even fruit purées, tinned fruit in fruit juice or dried fruits are fine. Also, the occasional square or two of good-quality 70% cocoa chocolate, biscuit or cake can top off a meal and satisfy a sweet tooth.

- Don't forget the snacks. Children are normally ravenous when they come home from school, and often can't make it between meals without something to eat and drink. Have healthy snacks to hand (see pages 110–111) and offer them regularly, as this will help to keep blood sugar levels stable, prevent cravings and overeating, and give your children something nutritious in place of the unhealthy snacks they may be eating now.

Putting it together

Let's look at some easy to prepare, healthy meals and snacks.

Breakfast

This meal is of the utmost importance in controlling weight and also, ironically, the one meal that kids often skip. While it is never a good idea to force kids to eat when they are not hungry, breakfast must be eaten, and this is something your children will need to accept. Most children will, once they begin a healthy eating programme, develop a more regular appetite, and be more refreshed and alert in the morning. So breakfast will eventually become more appealing – in fact, most kids will be ravenous for good nutritious fare.

Try to include a good source of protein – eggs, peanut butter, yogurt, milk, grilled lean bacon, or even cheese occasionally – in your child's breakfast. It will help to keep blood sugar levels stable throughout the morning, and aid concentration. As we learned in the previous chapter, children who eat a good healthy breakfast are far less likely to overeat throughout the day. Always add one or more servings of fruit as well – it gives them the nutrients they need to start the day well, plus it provides them with a healthy burst of energy to get them through the morning. Many kids will pick at fruit even if they are not natural breakfasters, so take this opportunity to squeeze in a couple of servings.

Ideas

- Healthy breakfast cereals are a great source of fibre, which aids digestion, is filling and encourages a sustained release of energy throughout the day. Porridge is a particularly good choice

- Make a breakfast buffet, with oatmeal, sesame seeds, sunflower seeds and dried fruits – such as apricots, raisins and cranberries – in small dishes. Each child can then create their own mixture

- Wholegrain cereal or muesli, sprinkled with seasonal berries or another fruit, with milk (try soya or rice milk occasionally to add variety) on top, along with a glass of juice – if the cereal needs to be sweetened, drizzle it with honey

- Wholemeal toast with peanut butter, a banana and a glass of juice

- Poached or boiled egg with wholemeal toast and a glass of juice

- Grilled lean bacon, a boiled egg, some berries or orange sections, a piece of wholemeal toast or muffin and some juice

- Plain yogurt (try soya yogurt as an alternative) with fruit (anything goes) and organic honey, a piece of wholemeal toast and a glass of juice

- A grilled lean bacon sandwich with tomatoes or cucumber on wholemeal toast, with a glass of juice

- Veggie sausage in a wholemeal bun, with fruit juice and an orange

- Fresh mango with yogurt, a handful of seeds or nuts, and a piece of wholemeal toast with butter or nut butter

- Wholemeal toast with pure fruit, low-sugar jam or preserve; yogurt (or a yogurt drink) and a glass of milk or juice

- Rice cakes with hummus, apple slices and juice

- A smoothie – fresh or tinned fruit, plain yogurt and honey whizzed together with a banana, or some ice cubes

- Grilled tomatoes, grilled mushrooms and grilled lean bacon with a slice of wholemeal toast and a glass of juice

- Or why not consider 'non-breakfast' foods, such as a tuna fish sandwich on wholemeal bread with a glass of juice? Or a leftover slice of 'healthy' pizza (see page 109)?

- If you are at a loss as to how to incorporate a few servings of fruit or vegetables, it's not hard. Some grapes on the side, or some orange, banana or apple sections are an easy choice. A pot of fruit in fruit juice, a few strawberries or other berries on cereal or yogurt, or whizzed into a smoothie, are other good ideas. Slices of cucumber, tomatoes or even pepper with bacon and eggs works well, too. A glass of pure fruit juice is also a whole serving of fruit, and you can normally encourage most children to drink a glass with breakfast. If you have a juicer, encourage your children to choose three or four fruits (kiwi, apple, mango, banana, pineapple, melon, for example) and add one vegetable, such as carrot, celery or cucumber, to add vital nutrients. A good simple combination for those new to juicing is apple and carrot – it's sweet, delicious and cheap.

Try to ensure that your child doesn't eat exactly the same breakfast every day – variety helps to ensure that he is getting the nutrients he needs, and also prevents further food fads from developing.

Lunch

With more and more children eating their lunch at school, many parents find it worrying that they have so little control over their child's diet during the day. But don't despair. Studies show that children, regardless of income, generally have higher intakes of key nutrients when they eat school lunch.

There has been a fairly major overhaul of school canteens over the past few years, and most schools now base their menus around government-recommended guidelines. There should, therefore, be more choice, as well as a greater number of fresh, whole foods available. If your child's school is the exception, find out why.

Many children eat better at school than they do at home because they mimic their peers. If a friend orders a previously untasted meal, other children will try it as well. And a hungry child is more likely to eat what's put in front of him, particularly if there are no alternatives available.

If your child eats at school, make sure he is aware of the basics of nutrition. Explain how a healthy meal will give him lots of energy for sports or tests in the afternoon, and how it will make him feel happier. As I pointed out previously, you can negotiate an eating plan that is acceptable to both of you – for example, at least two vegetables and one fruit at each meal (different ones every day, if possible), pasta, rice or wholemeal bread every day; and chips, ham and battered or deep-fried foods only once a week. If he knows the parameters, and knows that he can make the choices based on your agreement, he'll be more likely to stick to a healthy diet. Let him feel empowered rather than ruled. Show an interest in what he's eaten. Most children love reciting what they've had for lunch, right down to the last soggy Brussels sprout. Work out where the strengths and weaknesses are and base the rest of his daily diet on those. For example, if he's been short on fresh fruits and vegetables at lunchtime, serve a picnic tea with lots of fresh vegetables and dips, a platter of fresh fruit, yogurt, cheese and wholemeal toast. Even a bowl of fresh vegetable soup can make up for a less nutritious lunch.

Packed lunches

Lunchboxes give you a little more control over what your child is eating, although it's difficult to know what has been eaten if the lunchbox comes back empty every day. Many children simply tip out the contents rather than face an irate parent. The main solution is to discuss lunch in advance. Work out what your child wants and will eat, and try to incorporate that to some extent. Give them a list to choose from; for example, would you like egg salad, cheese and cucumber, tuna and sweetcorn, tomato and salad or peanut butter and banana tomorrow? Once again you'll be empowering them by offering choices, and children like to feel that they have some control over their lives. Children are also much more likely to eat something upon which they have decided.

The premise for healthy lunches is the same as for other meals. You want balance, nutrition, and a varied range of healthy foods (refer to the food pyramid on page 73). You also want to provide something that will actuallly appeal to a child, so that they'll be encouraged to eat it.

Ideas

• Fruit doesn't have to be fresh and raw to be nutritious. Little pots of tinned fruits in juice are also healthy and can be much more appealing to children.

• Peel oranges and tangerines before serving to make eating them easier (you may also want to choose varieties without seeds, as many kids dislike fruit because it has 'pips'). You can also cut up fruit, but dip it in a little lemon juice before wrapping to prevent discoloration. Dried fruit bars are also a good choice, and come in a variety of different flavours.

• Cut sandwiches into small bite-sized pieces that your child can pick up and eat while chatting to her schoolmates.

• Picnic-style lunches are always popular. Choose from small pieces of cooked chicken, yogurt, yogurt-based dips, fruit (such as grapes, cherries or strawberries), cheese, wholemeal pita bread, hummus, boiled eggs, raisins, dried fruits, raw vegetables (such as carrots, broccoli florets, olives, sliced cucumber, sliced peppers, celery and even a small pot of sweetcorn), unsalted nuts and rice crackers or cheese straws.

• Some children prefer to put together their own sandwiches – either at home before school, or at school, if you have supplied the makings.

- Hot meals – for example, leftover soups, stews or pastas containing some protein – can be kept hot in a Thermos. With a piece of fruit and a wholemeal roll, they'll have a completely balanced meal.

- For sandwiches, choose wholemeal bread or rolls over white, and include a source of protein (tuna, cold chicken, ham, lean roast beef, cheese, peanut butter or egg for example) to slow down the release of sugars into the bloodstream. Add some lettuce, cucumber, tomato or minced celery to the sandwich to make it more nutritious and to add some fibre, which has been shown to encourage a healthier weight.

- Try to avoid the crisp and treat trap – most kids' lunches these days consist of white bread sandwiches, a chocolate treat and crisps, which does not constitute a healthy meal in any shape or form. There is no reason to rule out crisps completely – you'd have full-scale mutiny on your hands! – but look for lower-salt brands, and agree to just one or two small packets per week (and that includes after-school snacks as well). You can also buy a large bag and give a few crisps a couple of days a week, in a plastic sandwich bag. Other alternatives include home-popped popcorn in a small bag, some trail mix (nuts, seeds and dry fruit), some cheese straws, rice cakes or mini rice cakes, low-sugar muesli bars, breadsticks or even dry cereal, such as plain Cheerios in a bag. In terms of something sweet, a small square of good quality chocolate won't do much harm or try a small packet of chocolate-covered nuts, raisins or sultanas, yogurt-covered raisins, dried fruit or fruit bars, a couple of biscuits wrapped up separately, or even a snack-sized chocolate bar, though once or twice a week only and only if the remainder of your child's lunch is healthy.

- Other good ideas to add to lunches are individual yogurts (squeezy ones are fine, but look for those that contain fruit and not chocolate, toffee or other sweets, and that are low in sugar and don't contain artificial sweeteners). Freeze them the night before so that they are still cold.

• Ask your child's school how they are supervised at lunchtime. Ensure that the children are encouraged to eat the healthy bits of their lunch before the treats, particularly if your child is a slow eater and some of his meal invariably comes home. Ask that the lunchbox is sent home unemptied so that you can see what has been eaten.

Hot lunches

Many parents worry that their children need a hot lunch, but this is simply not the case. A cold packed lunch can be just as nutritious, filling and low in fatty foods as a hot one. If your child does eat his main meal at lunchtime – at home, for example, or on the weekends – you can supply any of the dinner ideas (see page 112). Remember, two hot meals a day are not necessary, and many kids will end up taking in too many calories and fat if they have two heavy meals to contend with.

Super snacks

There are few children who can get through a day without a snack or two, and most school-aged children are encouraged to take one to school for break or recess. Snacks are important and, as I've said before, should never be dismissed as 'fillers' or inconsequential to a child's overall healthy eating plan.

If children are hungry, then by all means offer snacks. In fact, take it one step further and encourage your child to choose her own snacks from a 'snack drawer' or shelf in the fridge. She'll feel in control and will learn how to satisfy hunger with the appropriate foods. Do, however, put some rules in place: no snacks before meals, for example, and a maximum of three in an afternoon or five across a day. If you offer only healthy snacks, your child will eat healthy snacks. Children who learn to eat healthily when they are hungry (not when their parents say they are hungry) are more likely to learn good eating habits and self-control.

Encourage your child to consider whether or not she is really hungry. Some children eat because they are bored, or lonely, or even upset. Sometimes they cry 'hunger' when they want a little attention, or a treat. If they learn that hunger is satisfied by healthy

CHILD-FRIENDLY FOOD

There's no point in changing your family's eating habits only to find that your children will not touch a thing. Obviously hunger will set in eventually and they'll give in, but why not make it more fun.

First of all, children don't like to feel different. If they have chicken nuggets and chips at their mates' houses, they'll probably want the same at home. They might actually feel embarrassed about bringing friends home for dinner if stuffed peppers are on the menu. The thing is that it is possible to present healthy food in a way that will appeal to kids, and prevent them from feeling like social lepers.

Baked potatoes with cheese and baked beans alongside some crudités (cut up cucumbers, cherry tomatoes, carrots, sweetcorn and peppers) will appeal to most children, even faddy eaters. They don't have to eat everything on their plates. Allow them to choose – if you've put enough veg on their plate they'll choose some. Chicken legs baked in the oven with a little honey and served with mashed potatoes or rice and some kid-friendly vegetables (sweetcorn, peas and small broccoli florets) is normally acceptable for most kids and their friends. Alternatively, try a nutritious pasta, with tomato sauce, and throw in some vegetables or grate them in. Dip chicken fillets in egg and coat in organic wholegrain flour or wholemeal breadcrumbs and lightly fry in olive oil – better

foods, they will learn to eat only when they are hungry. And if hunger is no longer the cause of their discontent, they are much more likely to address the real reason why they wanted food in the first place.

The key to supplying snack foods that your child will eat is to make them easy, fun and accessible. Have a snack ready after school (even if you aren't there, you can have one waiting on a plate in the fridge, or ask your childminder or other carer to prepare one). If a hungry child comes home and you 'suggest' an apple, you may face objections. But if a sliced apple, a yogurt and a few raisins are already waiting on the table, they are more likely just to dive in and eat rather than complain. Peel oranges in advance and wrap them in Clingfilm; arrange crudités on a plate with some hummus or another dip, or set out breadsticks with a small pot of peanut butter for dipping. Make it look appealing and fun.

still grill – for homemade chicken nuggets or goujons. Chips can be easily made by parboiling sliced or chipped potatoes (try leaving the skin on) and then baking in a little olive oil in the oven. Oven chips are an acceptable second best, but choose those that are not 'coated', or prepared with hydrogenated vegetable oils. A homemade burger can be extremely nutritious if you use good-quality lean beef and serve it on a wholemeal bun. Add an egg, some ketchup, Worcestershire sauce, wholemeal breadcrumbs and pepper to the drained mince, mix and mould them into burgers. Bake or roast them for the healthiest burger. And healthier pizza, too, can be made at home using an organic flour tortilla as a base (or a wholemeal pizza base) and adding a little cheese, plenty of veggies and lean meat. Most kids will also eat some homemade chilli. Make fruit salads for dessert, or put together a yogurt and fruit 'bar' from which children can prepare their own deserts. You can also freeze yogurt or fresh fruit juices to make healthy ice-lollies.

It's not as difficult as you think! No child needs to feel that they'll be forced to exist on lentil curry. Certainly it's important to experiment with different foods, trying out new ones regularly, as well as introducing new flavours, tastes, textures and ingredients. You want to ensure variety and you'll want to expand your child's dietary horizons. But kid-friendly doesn't mean unhealthy. It's the way it's prepared and cooked, and what you serve it with, that makes all the difference.

Similarly, if you send in snacks for breaks at school, make them easy. Few children who want to spend their breaks playing will take the time to peel a tangerine. So peel and cut up fruit, put things in small bags for easy access, or choose low-sugar muesli bars or small packets of nuts or seeds that can be eaten quickly. Again, try to avoid crisps and chocolate for snacks. One thing we do have to do is to teach our children that these foods are not 'snack' foods, and that snacks are, really, little meals – and they must be healthy. On an occasional basis, as part of a healthy meal, these can be offered as a 'side' (for example, a few crisps on the side of a tuna sandwich, with some cucumber slices and carrot sticks will do no child any harm; or a small piece of chocolate after a piece of fruit for dessert is not a problem either), but not as a snack. If children get used to grabbing a packet of crisps or a chocolate bar for snacks, the weight will continue to pile on.

Snack ideas

• Fresh fruit or fruit salad

• Dried, unsulphured fruit or dried fruit bars

• Nuts (after the age of five, and if there are no allergies)

• Toast with peanut butter, yeast extract (but watch the salt content), cheese or a mashed banana

• Low-sugar muesli bars – particularly those with fruit and nuts

• A bowl of unsweetened cereal – dry or with milk

• Fresh popcorn (you'll need to supervise this) without salt or sugar

• Breadsticks (choose those with seeds, if possible)

• Rice cakes (preferably brown, spread with hummus, peanut or other nut butters, low-sugar fruit preserve, mashed bananas, Marmite or even a little butter)

• Yogurt (not chocolate, toffee or other 'dessert'-style yogurt; fruit and low-sugar or plain with added fruit and honey are best)

• A couple of good-quality biscuits (plain digestive biscuits or shortbread are OK in moderation, and contain fewer additives, salt and sugar than many brands) or crackers with cheese

• Hummus and pita bread

• Raw vegetables (for example, cauliflower and broccoli florets, peppers, celery, carrots, cucumbers, mange tout)

• 'Milkshakes' with fresh milk (better still, rice milk), a banana, some fresh fruit juice and a little yogurt. Freeze a couple of bananas to add to the blender to make the milkshakes creamy cold!

- Ice-lollies made from fruit juice (these are very inexpensive and easy to make, and you can add extra pieces of fruit to make them more filling; or mix with yogurt to make a creamy version)

- Homemade or good-quality cakes, such as carrot or banana (not every day of course but they're OK on a relatively regular basis as long as they don't contain a lot of sugar and are made with wholemeal flour)

- Cheese (good quality without additives and colourings)

- Small sandwiches on wholemeal bread – mini buns are ideal for this; it's interesting to note that a healthy sandwich with some lean meat, cheese and salad, or egg and cress, for example, can contain far fewer calories and fat than many of the typical snack foods that kids like.

 CASE HISTORY: **Kieron**

Kieron was a classic snack-food addict and although he ate normal, healthy meals with this family, his snacks were contributing to a serious weight problem. His parents encouraged him to keep a food diary to work out where the problem areas might be and it soon became clear that the fizzy drinks, chocolate bars, crisps and other snacks that he was buying from the school vending machine, and on the way home, were at the root of the problem. Rather than cut out snacks completely, he began to take a small sandwich for break time, and some fruit and muesli bars for after school. He still had the occasional packet of crisps or a chocolate bar, but he limited it to once a week (on 'health' reasons), and he always chose fruit juice or water over fizzy drinks.

It didn't take long for this change in eating habits to make a difference. Within a week his weight had stabilized, and over the next month he lost over a stone – eating as much as he ever had, but just choosing different foods. He was delighted by the change, and very surprised that his snacks could have been such a problem.

Dinners

Once again, these don't need to be heavy or hot to be nutritious. A salad with tuna or boiled eggs, some wholemeal bread and cheese, and some fruit is a great meal for kids – well balanced, nutritious and unlikely to lay down fat or lead to overweight. Plan your meals around as many fruits and vegetables as possible and you'll be off to a good start. Roasts are very easy to prepare and although many parents don't have the time to cook one before dinner in the evenings, you can cook them the night before and serve them cold, or warm them in the oven before serving. Roasts don't necessarily have to be accompanied by roasted potatoes doused in fat, or Yorkshire puddings and gravy either. Roasted meat, salad and fresh wholemeal bread is equally good. And the leftovers from a big roast can be used for soups, stews and sandwiches throughout the week.

Other ideas for dinners

• Grilled chicken breasts or roasted chicken legs with baked potatoes or new potatoes, green beans, broccoli and carrots

• Veggie sausages (some varieties taste great and they have far less saturated fat than meaty ones) with baked beans, rice or new potatoes and sliced cucumber

• Any roasted meat or poultry with steamed potatoes or rice and plenty of fresh vegetables (raw or cooked)

• Chilli con carne with rice or a baked potato and salad

• Spaghetti bolognese and salad or crudités

• Wholewheat pasta with a vegetable-based sauce and crudités

• Lean meat or poultry stir-fry, with honey and a little soya sauce, plus any combination of vegetables and rice

• Chicken strips, dipped in egg and then wholemeal breadcrumbs and grilled, with fresh vegetables and rice or potatoes

- A big bowl of vegetable soup with wholemeal bread, cheese and crudités

- Pork chops with apple sauce, roasted potatoes (parboil them first, drizzle with olive oil and roast) and any combination of vegetables

- Lasagne, substituting ricotta or cottage cheese for the béchamel sauce, and topping with only a little grated cheese, with salad (or crudités, which kids tend to like more)

- Roasted vegetables with couscous and crumbled feta cheese

- Turkey or chicken breasts grilled with lemon and herbs, and served on a wholemeal bun with crudités or salad

- Homemade burgers (see page 109) with crudités and homemade chips

- Homemade pizza (see page 109) with crudités

- Fajitas – strips of chicken, beef or turkey sautéed in a little olive oil with chilli seasoning, onions and peppers, and served in a wholemeal tortilla wrap with a little salsa

- Salmon fillets or tuna steaks, served with new potatoes and any combination of vegetables

- Fish pie – cod, prawns and tuna can be added to boiled potatoes and steamed vegetables and served in a sauce made from Boursin cheese (or another soft cheese made with herbs) and a little milk and stock. Top with sunflower seeds and bake

- Stews and casseroles with plenty of vegetables and lean meats, cooked with some wine, herbs and stock, which will naturally thicken when reduced. Serve with a wholemeal roll or rice, plus some salad

- Chicken cordon bleu – flatten a boneless chicken breast, place a slice of lean ham and a slice of cheese in the centre, roll and secure with a toothpick. Sauté lightly in a little olive oil to seal, and then bake in the oven until cooked, with a little white wine and stock. Serve with salad and rice. Kids love it and it's a low-fat version of breaded Kiev-type chicken dishes.

Desserts

There is no reason why a sweet ending is out of the question. If your child has eaten plenty of fresh fruits and vegetables throughout the day, and little or no sweet treats, it's certainly acceptable for them to have a small slice of cake or a brownie, a small bowl of ice cream or a few biscuits for pudding. As you'll discover later on in this chapter, restricting foods too heavily destroys the pleasure of eating and gives children no real understanding of balance. The key is to avoid offering extra, unnecessary treats between meals, or the same types of treats every night for dessert. Yogurt, rice pudding with sultanas, baked apples with raisins and a little brown sugar, fruit salad or fruit-based ice-lollies are healthy alternatives, and most kids will accept them without a murmur. You can even grate a bit of 70% cocoa chocolate over the top – you may be surprised to hear it but good-quality, dark chocolate is a rich source of iron and several trace elements. Because it doesn't contain the sugar levels of most confectionery, it doesn't affect blood sugar levels in the same way. And because it's rich, a little is more than enough!

Keep cream and sugar to a minimum when serving desserts. A bowl of fresh berries needs little or no sweetening – though you can dust them with icing sugar if they are particularly bitter. If fruit doesn't make up the bulk of the dessert, try to serve some fruit alongside so that children learn the importance of having healthy elements to their puddings. Tinned sliced peaches are a great topping for ice cream, a slice of pineapple on its own is a lovely treat, and mango can be cubed and served with yogurt and honey. On some nights just a banana or an apple, or some fruit tinned with fruit juice will be enough. Give your children some healthy options and let them choose.

What about fast food?

There is no doubt that if you deny your child fast food completely, it will be his first port of call when he has some money and the choice is his own. Unfortunately, fast food is part of our culture, but children have to learn that this type of food is not healthy and that it can be eaten only as a very, very occasional treat. But don't hesitate to teach your kids why – explain that a burger and chips constitutes the better part of a whole day's fat and calorie allowance, and that too much salt can be dangerous. Encourage them to choose fruit juice, milk or water to go alongside, instead of fizzy drinks. Choose thin-crust pizzas with vegetable toppings, and give the garlic bread a miss. Choose boiled rice over fried rice, and stir-fried vegetables and meats if you are going Chinese or Thai. Any other meals served that day should be fresh, low in fat, and based around fresh fruit and vegetables. You can also suggest that they take a good long walk, a swim or a run in the park to make up for the extra fat that fast food contains. Anything you can teach your child about healthy eating will work towards establishing healthier habits.

Convenience foods

There will be times, too, when a convenience meal from the supermarket is the only alternative. It's not the end of the world, either, as long as the majority of your child's diet is sensible. But think carefully about what you buy: thin-crust pizzas with vegetable toppings are far healthier and much less fatty than thick-crust, pepperoni pizzas with extra cheese; choose ready-made pasta sauces that have a lower sugar content; go for vegetable-based curries in light sauces rather than creamy alternatives and serve with plain rice and vegetables; opt for vegetarian burgers and sausages occasionally, which tend to be lower in fat and a good varied source of protein; choose chicken breast goujons over nuggets made out of 'reformed' chicken, and look for those with a lower fat content – better still, choose grilled chicken pieces instead. Balance your convenience offerings with fruit or yogurt for dessert, and fresh fruit juice alongside.

Remember, too, that there is no reason why a sandwich and a bowl of soup, or an omelette with salad, can't suffice on busy days. They are easy to prepare and certainly nutritious. Avoid creamy salad dressings where possible, skip the extra cheese or the garlic bread, and add some extra nutrients by including seeds and nuts in salads, sprinkled on pastas or served alongside stir-fries.

Getting kids to eat vegetables

Vegetables are the foods most likely to be shunned by children. However, there are many creative ways to encourage your children to eat and love vegetables. Children need to eat frequently and snacking is important, but they need to avoid nibbling or grazing on filling foods that are not nutrient-rich or filling up on juice or fizzy drinks. Making a snack of creatively-laid-out, appealing fruits or vegetables and serving them with healthy dips is a great solution.

When it's mealtime, serve vegetables as a first course 'appetizer' when kids are the most hungry; then add the rest of the meal after they've eaten the vegetables. Experiment with different sauces to make them taste better and be more fun. Almost everything tastes better with a sprinkle of lemon juice or a *little* butter. Explore and find a variety of vegetables and, when serving ones your children have never tried, get excited about them. Mash or cream veggies into stews or soups, grate them into sauces, and try juicing vegetables. Assume your child is going to love salads, greens and other veggies. Show them how much you love these wonderful foods. Set a great example by eating healthily yourself.

Get your kids involved with the growing, shopping and cooking of vegetables. Farmers' markets can be a fun shopping trip. Teach them what vegetables will do for their body and how important they are. Children are fascinated with and want to learn about their bodies. The more they learn the better choices they will make. Teach them to cook! If a child has made a salad, he's more likely to eat it – and the same goes or almost any other food! Ask every child to choose a vegetable and to prepare it occasionally (on a lazy Sunday, for example). Get a good kids' cookbook, and ask them to choose some healthy foods, list the ingredients for you to buy, and then make it themselves. Even very young children can help out in the kitchen – stirring, 'cutting' soft foods with a butter knife, or pulling the tops off strawberries, for example.

ENCOURAGING CHILDREN TO DRINK WATER

With the unbelievable range of brightly coloured, highly flavoured children's drinks on offer, it's not surprising that water ranks a poor second (or third, or fourth) with kids. There are, however, ways to introduce it fairly painlessly:

- Keep a jug of chilled filtered or bottled water within reach in the fridge. If it's the easiest drink to hand, they'll be more likely to drink it.
- Don't buy anything you don't want them to drink. In the end, if they are thirsty, they'll drink what's on offer.
- For hardened squash drinkers, gradually dilute the amount of syrup until they are drinking mostly water. They might complain, but they'll get used to it and the transition to plain water will be easier. Eventually stop buying it. If they want an alternative to squash, offer pure fruit juice diluted with water with meals only.
- If you have older children who drink too many fizzy drinks, explain the reasons why you are concerned (see page 32). Buy sparkling natural mineral water if they want something with a little fizz, and a variety of pure fruit juices to mix. For active kids, or aspiring sportsmen and women, explain that water is the best rehydrator there is – all the top athletes drink it.
- Consider investing in a watercooler, which can serve chilled purified water at the touch of a button. The novelty factor will persuade some children to drink more in the beginning, and it will soon become a way of life.
- Buy a plastic sports water bottle for each child, and keep it filled in the fridge. It will need to be washed and refilled daily to prevent a build-up of bacteria, but it can be theirs for the day – wherever they are.
- Set a good example. If they see you drinking Diet Coke with your lunch, they'll want some too. The whole family needs to convert if you want to succeed.

Most importantly, don't give up too soon. When trying to introduce new foods serve them at least five different times before giving up. Don't take the first 'no' for a final answer and think they'll never eat it again. You can even present it again shortly after it has been turned down. Do all this calmly and respectfully without nagging or bribing. Research backs up the fact that this can work. Several studies have found that repeated opportunities to sample new foods can alter a child's response from rejection to acceptance.

Faddy eaters

Herein lies the root of the problem facing many parents. It's very, very difficult to plan healthy, balanced meals when you've got children who refuse to eat them. Early in life, most children cotton on to the fact that their parents are concerned about how much and what they are eating. Making a fuss about food guarantees instant attention and many children slide into the habit of using food to wield power over their parents. Other children are simply not interested in food and the concerted efforts of their parents to make them eat put them off even further. For parents of all picky eaters, the best advice is to remove the pressure. If children fail to get a response, they get bored. If they realize that they won't get attention for eating badly, they'll stop using food as a tool to do so. If the pressure is off at the dinner table, children will start developing a healthier attitude to food – seeing it simply as something that is there to eat. It's neither poison nor is it a miracle medicine. Food can be enjoyed when it is not associated with parental nagging.

How can I change my child's eating habits?

Don't make a fuss at mealtimes. There will be times when your child is starving and will demolish anything in sight. At other times, they will pick and graze and seem to need nothing substantial. Go with the flow. Never force a child to clear her plate. She'll grow up associating food with stress and bad behaviour.

• If your child genuinely doesn't like something – mushrooms, for example – don't force it. Suggest that she tries one bite. If you're trying something new and she claims not to be very hungry, suggest three bites of everything on the plate. Children need to learn to try foods, and they need to eat a variety of good foods in order to stay healthy.

• Show some respect. We all have foods we don't like, and there are very healthy eaters who simply cannot abide a particular vegetable, meat or flavour. Don't force food that a child dislikes. The problem with faddy eaters, of course, is that they claim not to like anything. That's a different scenario. If your child eats well, tries new things and eats a healthy, varied diet, then the odd 'no-way' food can be dropped from the daily diet. But don't give up. Try new recipes. Introduce it again in a month's time. Children's tastes change and what may have been considered revolting one week may be the new favourite later on. If your child rejects a food after trying it a number of times, and continues to dislike it despite your best efforts, leave it for a period of time.

- Don't offer alternatives. Serve a healthy meal for the whole family and don't panic if your child doesn't eat much. If they are hungry, they will eat. Even the most resolute child will not starve himself to death.

- Invite a good eater round for dinner – often! Children like to do what their peers are doing, and if that involves eating new foods, they'll do it.

- Educate your child. Explain what foods are healthy and what they do for our bodies.

- Don't label your child. Parents often create self-fulfilling prophecies. If a child is accused of being picky, he will be. If you continually praise your child during meals for what they do eat, and insist to everyone around that your child is such a healthy eater, he'll take some pride in this achievement.

- Don't give up! Picky eaters are often picky because we allow them to be. If you give in and serve only what your child will eat, you will be setting up unhealthy eating patterns that can run through his whole life. Serve good healthy meals at every sitting. Offer the normal treats, and balance the good with the bad parts of his diet.

- Empower your child. If your child feels that she's lost control, she'll dig in her heels or revert to tears or tantrums. Make up a list of eight or nine good healthy meals, with a variety of different vegetables on the side. Let each child in the family choose a particular night's menu. You can suggest that there have to be at least four fruits or vegetables with every meal, and at least two have to be different from the meal chosen for the previous night. If you make it into a game, children will be more likely to be interested and become involved. They'll also feel that they have some control.

- Introduce new foods alongside the old favourites, and then slowly drop the parts of your child's diet that concern you most. Don't be tempted to launch a dramatically different eating programme overnight. You'll incite mutiny! Instead, make small changes. Every new food that your child eats is a step in the right direction.

- Introduce a star chart for younger children. They can be encouraged to put a star up for every healthy or new food they eat. When they reach an agreed total, you can offer a treat.

- If you have a grazer on your hands, make sure that the snacks he eats are nutritious. Some children just can't seem to stomach a big meal and prefer to eat little and often throughout the day. This style of eating is fine, as long as the foods eaten are nutritious and balanced. But whatever your child eats throughout the day, sit him down and make sure he eats it at the table. You don't want to encourage eating on the run, which can develop into a bad habit. If he's had plenty of small meals throughout the day, he won't want a big dinner, but serve smaller portions of whatever you are serving the rest of the family.

- If your child refuses food or just picks at his food, don't push it. Don't make your child feel guilty if he's just not hungry, and don't ever make him eat to please you. This sort of emotional blackmail can lower your child's self-esteem and make him insecure.

- Eat the same foods as your children. There should be no distinction between children's food and adult food. Good, healthy food is appropriate for the whole family. If children see their parents enjoying a broad range of foods, they'll be more likely to try some.

• Picky parents are more likely to produce picky kids. Try to expand your own diet to include foods that you don't normally eat. You might find that your tastes have changed, too. Don't only serve foods that you like. Try new recipes and be more adventurous. What you want to aim for is variety. If your child sees you eating something different, she'll naturally think she has the right to an alternative too.

Portion sizes

Keep them small! Children will never learn to moderate their own intake or learn when they are full if they get into the habit of clearing huge plates of food at every sitting. If they've had enough, allow them to say so. As long as they've eaten a reasonable quantity of the healthy food on their plates (including at least some vegetables), then let them be finished if they say they're full. If they are still hungry, respect their right to ask for more. Place serving dishes on the table and encourage kids to help themselves. Overweight kids might go a little mad at the outset, and fill their plates unnecessarily, but they will soon learn that there is plenty of food, no mad rush to finish it quickly and that there are no unhealthy foods on the table that will contribute to weight gain. As long as kids are encouraged to eat at least a little of everything offered, you can give them some free rein.

Never, ever insist that a child clears his plate. Again, a child will lose that important trigger mechanism that tells him when he is full. And there is plenty of evidence to back this up. For one thing, when parents try to control what and how much a child eats it can affect the natural mechanism that controls food intake – in other words, it can mean that they never learn self-control if they never let their bodies tell them when they are full. For example, a 1980 study found that when parents force children to clear their plates, those children may learn that the amount of food remaining on the plate is what matters, not the internal cues signalling hunger or being full. Given the growing problem with obesity, this is important. And part of this is also offering some choices – all healthy – so that they actually learn to choose to eat healthy foods if and when they are hungry.

Food restrictions

The point I made earlier about getting rid of the junk is important. If you regularly have such foods around and put tight restrictions on your child's intake, they may well develop an obsession. What needs to happen is that kids make choices from the wide range of healthy foods offered to them, so you don't need to regularly restrict foods. The importance of this is well documented. One study found that restricting access focuses children's attention on restricted foods, while increasing their desire to obtain and consume those foods. What this basically means is that if you fill your kids with healthy fare and offer the odd not-so-good foods on an occasional basis, they're much less likely to feel that they are doing without. This is another reason why it's so important that the whole family adopts a healthier diet.

Researchers have also found that highly controlling approaches to child feeding undermine children's ability to develop and exercise self-control over eating. Parental control in child feeding is negatively associated with preschool children's ability to self-regulate their energy intake.

Eating should be fun and rewarding. It's our job to provide wholesome, nutritious foods and their job to decide how much they want to eat. Kids will eat as much as they need. They will not let themselves go hungry. Meals should be relaxing and pleasant – nagging children to eat what you want them to does not work and is not respectful.

Eating together

One of the most important ways to implement a healthy eating programme and to keep tabs on what your child is eating is to sit down together as a family for meals. We've already discovered that eating together as a family is linked to lower weight in children, a higher intake of healthy foods, including fruits and vegetables, and greater self-esteem. It's also one of the most important ways that you can establish a healthy relationship with food. Children who eat alone never learn that meals are pleasant occasions, where people interact, try new foods together, share details of their day and enjoy the experience of discussing food – the way it's cooked, favourite combinations, ideas for different menus, likes and dislikes and even a little mimicry (trying foods that others find delicious). Children who eat only 'kiddie' food also never learn to expand their food repertoires and can end up being faddy eaters with unhealthy habits that last into adulthood. They don't learn to try new things, or to experiment. Kids whose parents sit over them and watch them eat feel under scrutiny and often use this to gain attention by making a fuss, developing fads and dislikes, making demands or even refusing to eat perfectly good food. They learn only to eat a small range of foods – those that parents insist they eat, or which they place in front of them – and never have the pleasure of sharing the experience. After all, meals are not just about clearing plates, eating to demand or swallowing healthy fruits and vegetables.

At the other end of the spectrum, kids who are left to eat alone or in front of the television don't pay attention to what they are eating or even how much. They don't recognize when they are full, because the process of eating has been overtaken by either a battle with parents, or the lure of a television programme. They may also make the wrong food choices with no-one to oversee what they are eating. Remember, too, that many overweight children are enormously conscious of their weight and feel embarrassed about eating 'in public'. This, of course, is a slippery slope, because once they start eating alone on a regular basis, there is little need for self-control and certainly no external control. Overweight children need to learn that there is nothing wrong with a healthy appetite; that everyone has to eat, whether they're slim or overweight, and that eating is not an embarrassing or compromising activity. By eating together, your overweight child will learn to feel less self-conscious about eating, particularly if you all eat the same foods and do not comment on any one family member's intake (or lack of intake). Also, if you are all eating the same things she won't feel that she is on a special diet, and will feel reassured that her meals are the same as everyone else's. Gradually the activity of eating will become less problematic and your child will develop a healthier relationship with food.

Interestingly, eating together with the family has been associated with improved school and psychological performance. And in two studies of school-aged children, frequency of eating family dinner was associated with increased discussion and knowledge of topics related to nutrition.

Make mealtimes fun with lots of conversation and laughter. Children are much more likely to eat what is placed in front of them – that is, healthy food as opposed to the sorts of treats they might previously have demanded – if there is no pressure to clear their plates and no intense focus on what they are eating. They will also learn to associate food with pleasure and fun and it will become less of an emotive issue.

It can be difficult to sit down together as a family, particularly if one or both parents work late. If you work, encourage your child's carer to sit down and eat with him. If you are at home with your kids, and want to eat with your partner much later, you can still sit down and have a little bit of what your children are eating. Sip a cup of soup or eat a salad later on. It's much healthier to eat earlier in the evening, to give your body a chance to digest the food before bed. Alternatively, give your children a nutritious 'tea', with fresh vegetables, fruit and maybe some toast after school. They can then last a little longer and eat a proper meal with you a little later.

Make an effort to have breakfast together. Rising a little earlier might not be a popular prospect for all family members, but it is important to at least attempt to eat as many meals as possible together. Your children won't be tempted to slouch off without eating anything – or cover their nutritious cereal with a mountain of sugar. They may also get over the hurdle of going without breakfast, and not being natural breakfasters, by simply taking part in a family activity rather than being the sole focus of a parent's attention – or ire! If it's part of the routine, kids will take part.

At the very least, ensure that some time is slotted in at the weekends for family meals. It's no good giving children a healthy meal and then shuffling them off to bed in order to have a takeaway with your partner. They'll feel let down and isolated, and also feel the food that you are feeding them is somehow inferior. That goes for treats, too – palming them off with a pizza and a video can certainly be an occasional treat, but they will never learn to try new foods if you aren't there to set an example on a regular basis.

The most important thing to remember is that there is no such thing as 'kids' food'. Food is food, and every family member should be eating the same things. It's an impossible pressure on most parents to produce two wholesome, separate meals every day, and rather than even try, we tend to choose the easy option and give the kids something quick and, very often, tinned or frozen. No child will ever grow up to enjoy a wide variety of foods or have a clue about nutrition if they are fed the same unhealthy foods every day.

That does mean choosing foods that the whole family will enjoy, but look at this process as a pleasurable one. Kids can have some great – if somewhat eccentric – ideas about what foods go well together, and they'll enjoy playing some part in the menu planning as well. I speak from personal experience here. I used to sit my children down to eat early, in order to get them to bed at a reasonable time. I served them healthy, nutritious meals, but they did tend to have a sort of tedium to them and, in an attempt to avoid the meal-time battle, I focused on the foods they liked to eat. When I was divorced, I started eating with them at the earlier time, and because there was no way that I was going to survive on their limited repertoire, I changed tack completely and simply served them whatever I fancied. They were very doubtful at the beginning, and horrified to find that some of my favourite foods were a) bright green (Thai curry), b) spicy and c) full of every vegetable combination under the sun. Children don't eat Thai food, they chorused (although I could neatly sidestep that one by pointing out that Thai children certainly did). But they learned to adapt. They added fromage frais (sometimes even the fruity type) to cool down the spicy foods, or apple purée to 'sweeten up' the vegetables they weren't particularly fond of. They came up with some great ideas to make the food taste better (to them), and some combinations that I might never have thought of. Cauliflower cheese with vegetables on the side became cauliflower, broccoli, spinach and cheese because they preferred all the vegetables to be mixed into the sauce – and it tasted delicious.

Give your kids a chance to become involved. If they develop a good relationship with food at an early age, they'll avoid the faddy eating traps that can lead to overweight, and eat the kinds of foods that keep weight problems at bay. Plus both you and they will benefit from the social experience of mealtimes, and begin to see food not as something problematic but as the happy reason for sitting down together and sharing time. Given the fact that so many overweight children have some emotional issues with food, this can only be a step in the right direction.

Using common sense

Don't be alarmed if you have a bad day, or even week. It's the overall balance that counts, not the daily or even weekly load. As adults, too many of us are used to diets that we slip onto and off of at random. You know the familiar scenario – you blow the diet by eating a chocolate doughnut and decide to start again tomorrow. Eating well is a way of life, not a diet, and it should be adopted permanently. The odd slip, treat, chicken nugget, chocolate bar or even packet of biscuits will not make a difference in the long term if you adopt an overall policy of healthy eating. The more good food there is in your child's diet, the less these slips matter.

Most importantly, however, eating well means changing our approach to food. As families we need to learn about food and the effects it has – both negative and positive – on our bodies. A healthy attitude is as important as healthy food, and we need to want what is best for our minds and bodies now and in the future. Cutting out crisps for a week is not going to make a substantial difference in the long term. Even if the changes are gradual, they must become an accepted way of eating – and an important part of our children's lives. It is never too late, nor is it too early, to start taking steps towards optimum health and well-being.

And remember – no diets!

The food you serve your children should be the food that the whole family eats – it should be tasty, nutritious and healthy, with as few as possible of the foods that we know cause obesity and overweight. The whole point of a healthy eating programme is to ensure that your children learn to eat good foods, and carry on doing so throughout their lives. If it's a short-term 'fix', 'diet', or solution, and you revert instantly to your old habits, your children will learn nothing, and any weight lost will eventually be regained. A healthy diet does include treats, the occasional fast-food experience and the odd packet of crisps or a chocolate bar. No-one is immune to the temptations of unhealthy treats, but as long as they are eaten in the context of an overall healthy diet, and eaten only minimally, there is nothing wrong with including them from time to time. No-one feels like they are missing out, or develops cravings for foods that are available occasionally. But most importantly, cravings for junk food and treats do tend to disappear – or at least be minimized – when our children are full, have a balanced diet with all the nutrients they need, are well watered and understand the importance of eating well. If you put a child on a diet, he instantly feels different, under pressure and restricted, which will ultimately backfire. Make it clear that the changes to your family diet are for health reasons – and make sure everyone is involved (see page 130 The Object of Eating Well).

Ultimately food is for eating – there are healthy foods and there are those that are less healthy. Children need to learn that no food is 'bad', but that there are some foods that need to be eaten in moderation because they make us fat and unhealthy. The key is to encourage your children to eat a broad range of different foods, to fill up on healthy offerings and to understand the concept that meals are pleasurable, social occasions, not eaten in solitude in front of the television, and that eating is a fun experience.

Teaching your children about nutrition

As adults, we can do a lot to guide them in the right direction. Educating them about food is an important part of this. I'm not suggesting nutrition lessons every Friday evening – simply explain what you are cooking or choosing at the supermarket and why. It means pointing out, whenever you get the opportunity, why some foods are healthier than others.

Children love information, and they'll feel important if you take the time to explain things. What's more, they won't feel completely alien when faced with friends who eat unhealthily and apply peer pressure. They can explain their choices and maybe even bring a few friends round to the concept as well. If a child can actually say

TOO BUSY TO COOK?

As we have already discovered, it doesn't take a lot longer to prepare nutritious, healthy meals than it does to pop some trays in the oven or the microwave. Obviously not all parents are natural cooks, and coming up with new ideas can be daunting. Furthermore, time constraints can make the process all that much more difficult. Here are some ideas to help make it work:

• Stick to a bowl of nutritious soup and a sandwich on wholemeal bread, with some fruit, cheese and crudités if you are busy; meals don't have to be complicated to be nutritious.

• If you have time on the weekend to cook a roast lunch, make a little extra of everything and freeze it.

• When you do make pasta sauces, soups, stews, casseroles or even chicken or meat dishes, double or triple the recipes and freeze them for busier periods.

• Stick to healthy old standbys, such as jacket potatoes with baked beans and cheese, or spaghetti with pesto and salad. Throw a handful of vegetables into the spaghetti water at the last minute to toss in with the pesto, to add some valuable nutrients to your meal. Even frozen fish fingers, made from cod fillet rather than pieces of reconstituted fish, in wholemeal breadcrumbs with a few oven chips is not an unhealthy dish. Try to find organic products, which must, by

that she is choosing juice over fizzy drinks because she likes the taste and because it doesn't make her fat, she's at least got an argument. If you ban fizzy drinks without explaining why, your children genuinely won't understand the reason why they are not on the family menu and indulge whenever they can.

Don't assume that they won't be interested. Teaching kids doesn't mean boring them with facts about vitamins and minerals. Make it relevant – if they're into football, point out that unrefined carbohydrates will give them more energy for the big match. If they've got a cold, explain that fresh fruits and vegetables have lots of vitamin C, which will help get rid of their cold. If they are constipated, explain that their diet is lacking some fibre or water or fruit and vegetables. You'll find lots of resources that can help you with this (see pages 249–261).

law, contain no unhealthy additives, and tend to have lower quantities of salt and other unhealthy ingredients, and make the meal complete by adding lots of vegetables (frozen will do), plus some raw baby carrots, celery sticks, cherry tomatoes and cucumber slices.

- Consider a big bowl of porridge; a bacon, tomato and lettuce sandwich on wholemeal bread; or an omelette or scrambled eggs. A favourite last-minute dish in our house is a spin on eggs Benedict: poached egg and lean ham on a toasted wholemeal muffin, with a sprinkling of cheese on the top and a crunchy side salad. And it's ready in less than 10 minutes – or as long as it takes to toast the muffins and poach the eggs. Any of the meals suggested earlier – for lunch or breakfast – are nutritious enough to take the place of dinner. Don't be bound to any rules that state dinners must be hot or big!

- And, as I've said before, don't feel bad if you have to resort to the occasional takeaway pizza. Make a wise choice – sticking to minimum cheese, thin crusts and veggie toppings, for example – and offer some crudités and fresh fruit on the side. Giving in to the occasional convenience meal doesn't mean you have wrecked your diet – because you aren't on a diet! Just make up for it the next day by serving something more wholesome, and less fattening or filling.

Most older children and teenagers want to know how nutrition can help them now. If you can convince teenagers, particularly those that are interested in sports, or taking exams, that food is fuel and that proper fuel will make a difference in their life today, you will be more likely to succeed in interesting them. Emphasizing the link between sports or exercise and food is a good plan. Nearly half of all adolescents are involved in at least one organized school sport or after-school activity. For teenagers who are inactive, the challenge is to convince them of the importance of both exercise and proper nutrition in developing a fit mind and body.

Active adolescents do best when they fuel their bodies with a high-energy diet based on the food pyramid. By emphasizing a diet full of carbohydrate-rich grains, fruits and vegetables, with a balance of lean protein foods and healthy dairy products, the body will be

THE OBJECT OF EATING WELL

Health is the first and most important object of changing your family diet. A family that eats well and takes regular exercise will, in the large majority of cases, simply not suffer from weight problems.

It is vital to remember that healthy eating is not a short-term solution, nor is it a 'diet'. It represents a change in eating habits that must become just that – habit. There are no quick-fix answers to a weight problem – the number of failed dieters around is testament to that. You must be prepared to commit to a better way of eating, and to stick to it regardless of other demands on your time and energy.

Children should not, under any circumstances, be placed on a weight-loss diet. **The aim of changing eating habits is to maintain weight until your child grows into it.** Some children do lose weight when their eating habits change, particularly if they were very poor eaters, heavy snackers, comfort eaters or simply constant grazers, but losing more than 0.5 kg (1 lb) or so a week is not recommended, and you will have to make sure that your child is eating enough to grow and develop properly.

The main difference between overweight adults and overweight children is the fact that children are still growing. Overweight adults do need to lose weight for health reasons and because they have stopped growing, their intake can be cut fairly dramatically without compromising their future health. That's not to say that dieting is recommended for any age group because, as we've seen already, diets don't work. Only broadscale changes to eating habits that are consistently maintained will have an effect. But it's very important that both you and your children understand that you are not changing your eating habits to see the figures on the scale go down. If you can keep weight stable as your child grows, you are doing exactly what is required. Your child will grow into his weight.

If your child is very dangerously obese, you may need extra help to ensure that gentle weight loss is maintained alongside growth (see Chapter 7). However, a change to healthy eating will result in a natural weight loss if that is what is required. Kids need plenty of regular meals and healthy food to grow and develop properly, to maintain mood, body functions, concentration and overall health. Restricting food will not only have an emotional impact and lead to further, unhealthy eating habits, but it can also damage your child's health.

Remember: while a child is still growing, the aim of treatment for obesity is to slow the rate of weight gain. Never reduce your child's food intake to promote weight loss without first consulting a doctor.

tuned for peak performance. Explain that during exercise carbohydrates fuel working muscles by breaking down glycogen, the storage form of carbohydrates which release glucose during muscle work. The body also relies on a steady stream of blood glucose to keep all body systems working effectively – including the brain. The more active the teenager, the more carbohydrates are needed. Is your child a budding athlete? Explain the concept of 'burn-out' and lack of stamina, which indicate that body carbohydrate stores are low. If you make healthy eating part of their language, they'll be much more willing to listen. In fact, you may find them taking some pride in adopting the diet of an athlete or a chess whiz. More often than not, they'll pass on the information to friends.

Remind your child that when it comes to brain power, eating a balanced breakfast every day is important. Good-quality food translates into better concentration and ability to learn. If your teenager is struggling with exams, or feeling stressed by the competition at school, offer some practical nutritional guidance. Dietary changes can be one of the greatest factors in overall success at school.

And not a mention of the word 'diet' or 'obesity'. If your child is overweight and concerned about the problem, you can explain how different foods contribute to weight gain, and show that as a family you understand the importance of maintaining a healthy weight. No child needs to be singled out for a lecture on foods he can and can't eat. The best way to go about changing children's eating habits is to educate them about the positive effects of healthy food and a healthy diet. When their weight starts to balance out, it will all begin to make sense.

Take them to the supermarket and show them food labels. Compare good and bad labels and look appropriately shocked at the labels for junk food. Let them feel that they are part of your programme. Enlist their help and ask their advice. Encourage them to choose fresh produce – teach them, for example, to look for firm cucumbers, and how to tell if a melon is fresh by its scent.

Avoiding the lure of advertising

This is all very well, you might think, until your child is bombarded with advertisements for unhealthy foods that look unbelievably appealing – and 'essential' for any 'cool' kid to eat or drink. There is a way round this. As I pointed out in Chapter 2, you need to educate your kids about advertising (see Resources page 253). Try to sit down and watch TV with your child. Point out why an advertisement is so successful – wow, you might say, they actually make crisps look healthy! Or that makes you want to buy it, doesn't it – even if we know it's not healthy? Take the opportunity to explain why some foods are not good for us – they're high in salt, fat, sugar, etc. – and how too much of these foods can make us fat, tired, moody and unhealthy. Engage your child's support, and ask him to tell you why something that looks appealing in an advertisement really isn't good. Children today occasionally read papers and catch a little of the news so they might be up on some current events. The trend towards obesity can't have passed them by, and if they have a weight problem themselves, you have an obvious opening to discuss some of the issues – for instance, 'All those ads make kids want to eat foods that make them fat'. You don't have to single your child out for special attention – make them understand the scope of the overall problem and some of the causes.

What next?

You'll notice the difference in your child's overall health when you change your family's diet. You will also notice a change in weight – that is, your child will stop gaining weight and may even lose some. But remember, diet is only part of the problem with the current trend towards obesity. If children aren't active, even a healthy diet can't keep overweight completely at bay. It will make a difference, but it's not the whole answer. Ultimately, fitness is part and parcel of a healthy lifestyle. And children who are active can enjoy more food without worrying that it will make them fat. What's more, the occasional treat or fast-food meal is never a problem when a child has a healthy diet *and* an active lifestyle.

Have you got a couch potato on your hands? In the next chapter, we'll look at how to get them moving.

Chapter Five

Exercise and Leisure

The importance of fitness can't be underestimated in the battle to curb the obesity trend. As we saw in Chapter 2, kids are simply not active enough to sustain the amount they eat. They walk less, take part in fewer after-school and in-school sports and activities, and leisure time seems to consist of plonking themselves in front of the television, computer or games console. Even with friends, activities tend to centre on the sedentary.

This is an obvious change from the type of upbringing most of us had, when we walked to and from school and then went straight out to play – on bikes or to the park, armed with a ball, some chalk to play hopscotch, or a skipping rope. Kids were inventive – they played 'it' and hide 'n' seek in groups; they made up games in nearby fields, parks or even woods; they walked there and back and had fun while doing so.

Today, of course, there are fewer parks, fields or woods in walking distance, and most facilities that are laid on by councils tend to be expensive and require parental accompaniment. Letting children play on the streets is hardly an option either. The increased number of cars and buses on the roads means that accidents are more common, so it's no longer safe for kids to play ball on the street, or ride their bikes together. Parents feel obliged to take their children out for exercise, which naturally means that it tends to be at a parent's convenience, rather than a natural occurrence. And because parents are busy and tend to get inadequate exercise themselves, it's all too easy for children to stagnate in front of the television or potter around the house. To compound matters, many parents fail to set good examples themselves. According to a 1999 survey, eight out of 10 of us get no regular exercise, so it's not surprising that our children are less active. Even very small children, who should be naturally active, are spending far too much time in sedentary pursuits.

Exercise reduces weight and keeps it under control for a variety of reasons, but it also helps to prevent many of the health and emotional problems associated with overweight. Let's look at what research tells us.

The benefits of exercise

- Exercise strengthens the cardiovascular system and increases heart mass. This reduces the risk of heart disease. Most studies concentrate on adults, but we do know that sedentary adults have a 30–40 per cent higher risk of death from coronary heart disease than those who exercise three to four times a week. Because the early signs of heart disease are becoming much more prevalent in children, it's fairly clear that exercise is necessary to reduce damage and prevent heart problems before they set in.

- Exercise helps to increase the metabolic rate – the rate at which our bodies burn calories. Exercise can burn enough calories to reduce body fat, leading to weight loss in those who are overweight. Obviously the degree of weight loss is dependent on the level and type of activity.

- Exercise dilates the blood vessels so that the heart can pump more easily to supply blood to the rest of the body. The result is that blood pressure declines. High blood pressure is on the increase in children – partly because of their inactivity, but also because of their high-fat, high-salt diets.

- Exercise reduces stress. Children and young adults can be exposed to a variety of stresses that can affect their behaviour and physical and mental health. Exercise works by using up the adrenalin that is created by stress and stressful situations. It also creates 'endorphins', the feel-good hormones that improve mood, motivation and even tolerance to pain and other stimuli. This may sound irrelevant to the average overweight child, but bear in mind that kids with weight problems tend to be the victims of teasing and bullying, and to have lower than average self-esteem (see pages 170–174).

- Exercise is good for the brain. Aerobic exercise helps to increase the number of brain chemicals called neurotransmitters, so that messages can be carried more quickly over brain cells. This increases mental flexibility and agility over longer periods of time. Furthermore, regular exercise increases the supply of oxygenated blood to the brain, which can improve concentration, alertness and intellectual capacity. Many overweight children feel sluggish, lethargic and tired a good proportion of the time, which affects their grades and, through that, their confidence and self-belief.

- Regular exercise can promote good, regular sleeping habits. Many children are simply not tired at the end of the day, which pushes bedtimes later and causes disrupted sleep (see pages 164–166). Children who are over stimulated by television, video games or too much homework may suffer a similar fate. Children need to experience physical exhaustion before they will settle down at an appropriate time and get a good night's sleep.

- Several studies show that children who exercise regularly are more apt to exercise when they become adults. This is important. Overweight kids are much more likely to become overweight adults unless their unhealthy lifestyle and eating patterns are changed.

- Regular exercise significantly enhances the body's ability to move air into and out of the lungs, increases blood volume and helps blood become better equipped to transport oxygen. This increases energy levels, which are often low in overweight kids. Having a bit more energy can inspire them to make the changes necessary to get their weight under control.

- Regular exercise reduces calorie intake. In a study of 43 overweight eight- to 10-year-old boys who attended a four-month programme consisting of one or two physical education sessions each week, daily caloric intake spontaneously decreased by 12 per cent. So not only does exercise burn off excess calories, but kids who exercise regularly are more likely to eat less.

- Preliminary evidence suggests that exercise helps to increase insulin sensitivity and resistance to diabetes. Studies indicate that more active individuals have a 30–50 per cent lower risk of developing diabetes than their sedentary peers. Exercise has been shown to delay or possibly prevent glucose intolerance turning into diabetes and also has benefits for those who are already diagnosed with diabetes.

- Exercise is now linked with self-esteem and mental attitude. Regular exercise produces muscle strength, gains in aerobic fitness, feelings of control over our environment and positive feedback from others, all of which can make children feel better about themselves. With self-esteem taking a battering in most overweight children, and depression and moods linked to the onset of overweight, this can be very important.

How much exercise do children need?

Before examining various ways to fit exercise into your child's lifestyle, it's important to assess just what physical needs children really have. In April 2004, the UK government issued guidelines suggesting 45 minutes to 1 hour of exercise for children, five days a week. These recommendations are, of course, nowhere near to being met by today's children, as we discovered in Chapter 2.

What type of exercise?

Children need the same types of exercise as adults – that is, exercise that promotes flexibility, builds muscle, gives the heart and lungs a good workout (aerobic) and makes them stronger. That doesn't mean heading down the gym every night. The majority of these needs can be met by playing, which is how children have always stayed fit and healthy. What we need to do, however, is to ensure that children are given the time and space to play, and the room to run! Let's look at some ideas:

- Large-muscle groups are worked by a variety of fun activities, including walking, climbing, gymnastics, kicking (a ball, preferably!) and skipping. These activities are also aerobic, providing they are undertaken for long enough (about 15 minutes).

- Aerobic exercise is best for the cardiovascular system. The most suitable aerobic activities for kids include swimming, skating, cycling, running, active team sports (football is an excellent example) and rollerblading.

- Exercises that improve and increase flexibility include tumbling (gymnastics), judo and karate, playground fun (hanging from climbing frames is ideal) and ballet. There are even yoga classes for kids, which can be great for stress reduction and grace.

- Your child will become stronger by taking part in any activity that uses his muscles – pushing and pulling on playground apparatus, swinging (which works the leg muscles), climbing and other activities such as running and skipping. Since muscle burns more calories than fat, by increasing your child's muscle mass, it can make it easier for him to lose weight and/or maintain a healthy weight.

- Go for sports that involve hand-eye (or foot-eye) co-ordination, including throwing and catching, baseball or rounders, cricket, football, tennis or squash – all of which improve grace, skill and, naturally, co-ordination.

- And don't forget to let them rest. For every 15 minutes of activity, children need to rest. You'll probably find that children wind down naturally. Watch a child in the park – he'll run and jump for about 10–15 minutes and then take a self-imposed break. Rest doesn't mean stopping activity altogether – reducing the intensity is often adequate – and it's not a good idea to flop in front of the TV, which can lead to sore or stiff muscles. Offer plenty to drink during rest periods.

• You must also allow a little time for cooling down. If your child is just out for a run in the park, or cycling, he'll wind down and hence cool down naturally. If he takes part in competitive sport, however, or anything aerobic, he will need to undertake some stretching exercises, and a little light jogging, to prevent injuries and stiffness, and literally 'cool down' the muscles.

Physical activity should be built into regular routines and playtime for children and their families. Additionally, physical activity should be done at an intensity that causes the child to breathe hard (mild discomfort), but not to the point of pain. If your child is normally sedentary, then physical activity should be started gradually.

It's important that children are involved in a variety of activities that make their bodies move. In fact, a recent study suggests that variety may be a helpful tool in keeping kids motivated. There is no need to sign your children up for the nearest aerobics class (unless, of course, that is of particular interest to your child). Children can get physical activity through active play, leisure-time activities and even household chores. Do, however, consider how appropriate the activity is to your child's age. For instance, according to the Nemours Foundation in the US, competitive sports are usually considered appropriate beginning between the ages of eight and 12, although it's certainly acceptable for kids to compete and train at younger ages as long as they are in the hands of an experienced coach.

Fitting it in
• First and foremost, you'll need to assess your schedule. If time is a problem, you may need to book 'fun' appointments for your children, to ensure that they are getting playtime. Given some freedom and a little open space, most children will get plenty of exercise with little prompting from their parents.

CASE HISTORY: ## Freddie

Freddie was 10 when his weight problem began to bother him. With Freddie's agreement, his parents changed his diet – and that of the whole family – to include foods that were lower in fat, salt and unhealthy junk. The aim was not weight loss, but health. He chose snacks for school that looked similar to those his friends were eating (bags of popcorn, instead of crisps, for example), but the real eye-opener for him was exercise. Freddie had always been an active boy, taking part in clubs and sports at school, but he was now finding that his weight was beginning to slow him down. The solution was to start taking the train to school instead of getting a lift, which meant a 20-minute walk to the station, both in the morning and after school. His parents also suggested that he take 30 minutes to do some sort of exercise every day – playing tennis with his mum, swimming, kicking a ball around with his brother or dad, or anything that got him up and going. He stuck to this religiously. Over the following year he grew substantially while maintaining the same weight, and he now looks and feels 'normal'.

• Make sure that your children get fun time every day. If it means turning them out into the garden, or making a visit to the local park, playground, swimming pool or gymnasium every day after school, you'll have to allow time. Try to remember that exercise is as essential as nutritious meals when it comes to overall health and battling a weight problem. Excuses won't wash.

• If your kids are very busy with school work or have a long journey home, or you don't get in until later, you'll have to adjust your schedule. Exercise doesn't have to be formal to be effective. In fact, studies show that walking is as good as any exercise in terms of weight control. Take a walk as a family in the evenings on busier days, or slot in an hour after dinner for leisure pursuits.

• Make sure that playtime takes place before homework. While it is tempting to 'clear the decks' when children get home, they will be tired from a day at school and will perform more efficiently after they have had some energizing exercise and probably something light to eat. Let them run off the steam that has built up over the school day. It will reduce stress levels and ease any tension that has built up.

• Don't rely on structured activities too much. While these are undoubtedly good for fitness levels, they can mean a lot of waiting around and are less useful for releasing built-up energy. Sometimes children just need to run and play, left to their own devices and without strict supervision.

• But do try some organized sports. Children need to have a flavour of all types of activities before they can decide what they like best. Don't be concerned if your child is not a natural athlete, and never criticize or suggest quitting, particularly if your child enjoys a sport. Team sports teach many things above and beyond fitness, and your child will benefit from a group activity. Many children begin sports in childhood that become hobbies in later life, so it's important to find something that they enjoy and will want to practise regularly.

• If the weather precludes outdoor activity, arrange some indoor games – running up and down the stairs, playing tag in a suitable room or even helping with the housework are all better than sitting still. You can be certain, however, that most children are undaunted by wet or cold weather. If they are dressed properly, they'll have as much fun in inclement weather as they will when it's sunny.

• Try to plan some family activities that involve exercise. After dinner, suggest a family walk around the block or a bike ride in the park. At the weekends, try to get out together with a visit to the park, woodland or zoo, the local swimming pool or gym club, or even the country, where you can spend the day in the fresh air. Everyone in the family will benefit from regular exercise, and you'll teach your children how to be active in their daily lives. For example, if they are used to 'burning off their dinner' after a heavy meal, they'll be more likely to adopt this habit in later life. Even city excursions or trips to a castle or funfair involve moving which is, again, much better than sitting in front of the computer or television.

• Make exercise fun (see page 142). If they think it's healthy, children will be unlikely to be enthusiastic. They'd probably say no to a chocolate bar if you called it healthy, so be prepared for resistance to doing what's good for them. Find activities that everyone enjoys and make them a normal part of your routine. Dragging kids away from the playstation for a jaunt in the park is unlikely to excite the average child. However, if you always go the park after school, or before Sunday lunch, they'll accept it as a natural part of life. Try a variety of different activities to keep up their interest, and, above all, make sure they enjoy it (see page 145 for some tips on nudging lazy children into action).

• Focus on the positive. If your child worships a particular athlete, point out how they train and become fit. You'll be much more likely to inspire a child into action if you can relate it to something with which she identifies.

• Join a gym that has children's activities. Many clubs now have programmes for children on the weekends, and you can go for a swim or take a class yourself. Many local community centres also offer the same facilities and are a good deal cheaper.

• Set a good example. If your leisure time involves a glass of wine and the newspaper, your children are unlikely to think that riding a bike is a normal weekend activity. Try not to groan and moan when they want to head to the park for a ball game, or suggest a swim. If you are enthusiastic about exercise, and become involved as much as possible, they will respond with equal fervour. Most of all, they'll enjoy your company, and feel reassured that you are interested in their interests.

• If walking to school or the local playgroup is impossible, park further away than usual and walk part of the way. Consider organizing a 'walking bus', which involves children walking to school in a large group, accompanied by a 'driver' (a parent volunteer at the front of the bus) and a 'conductor' (at the back of the bus). The bus stops at prearranged points to collect other children, who join the queue. (For further information on such schemes see Resources page 254.)

• If it's manageable, consider accompanying your child to school on bikes. Enrol your child in a cycling proficiency programme first, which teaches the basics of road safety, signalling and skills. Invest in a good helmet and a neon bib.

• Join in with fun runs and sponsored sporting events as a family.

Whatever you choose, make a decision to commit to it. As adults we are often wary of the term 'exercise' as it calls up visions of enforced routines at school, or hours on a treadmill trying to lose unwanted weight. Exercise holds no such associations for children, and we want to ensure that it never does. If they start off being active, they'll be more likely to continue that way. Early on we need to plant the idea that exercise is fun and sociable, it makes us feel better and, above all, it's a natural, normal part of life.

Making exercise fun

Stuck for ideas about how to encourage inactive children? Try some of the following:

• Change the name. If the idea of a walk does not excite your children, call it something else. Turn it into a game: a treasure hunt, for example. Get a local street map and ask each child to plan a different route each day. Or flip a coin at the end of every street to decide whether you will turn left or right (it may turn out to be a very long walk indeed). Go on a spying mission, where children are encouraged to find 10 different objects (all red, for example) before you can return home. Do your shopping locally and give each child a list of things they need to remember to get. If they feel that they have a mission, they'll be much happier to be involved.

- Start a get-fit campaign and make it fun. Children are enormously motivated by a little competition and if they see results, they'll be even more keen. My son's school set up a programme to improve the fitness of the boys. The children were evaluated for fitness levels and underwent a fitness improvement programme, with regular testing to assess the results. The vast majority of children were enormously motivated by this project – partly because of the competition element, but partly because they could see for themselves what exercise could do. This type of programme can easily be undertaken at home. Invest in a stopwatch and time your children running in the park, or around the block, even up and down the stairs. Write down the times on a chart and encourage them to better their results. How many sit-ups can they do in a minute, for example. Set up an obstacle course in the garden or a local park and time how long it takes to get round.

- Dance! Turn on the CD player and get the whole family involved. Dancing is great aerobic exercise and any musical activity can be uplifting. Make up your own line dances, or show your children how to jitterbug or tango. You might learn some more modern dances yourself. Allow your child to choose the songs.

- Create your own exercise video. If you have a video camera, it can be great fun to prepare a homemade exercise programme to music. Not only will the children have a good time (and get lots of exercise) while putting it together, they might be encouraged to use it themselves on a rainy day.

- Make up a game. Ask your children to come up with ideas for ball games, hopping or skipping games – or anything active. The idea is to keep moving, whatever inspires them.

• Walk the dog. Dog owners have much higher fitness levels than any other pet owners, and for good reason. All dogs need regular daily walks, and it can be the type of enforced exercise that becomes a healthy and enjoyable habit. If you don't have a dog, perhaps your children can offer to take a neighbour's dog for a daily walk in the park. Or perhaps you could just have your neighbour's dog round to play in your garden for a few hours a week – only if it's a saint with children of course.

• Set up a water park in the garden, with a slide, the sprinkler, some buckets, an inflatable pool and even the swing set. Ask your children to design the park so that there are lots of different activities on offer and then invite round some friends.

• Buy a packet of balloons and use wooden spoons or tennis racquets to play games in the garden. Set up a net with some string or use your garden furniture as the barrier. This game can also be played indoors, using kitchen chairs as a 'net'. If the kids are outside, fill the balloons up with water and get them to throw and catch the balloons without breaking them!

• Try to plan holidays with plenty of outdoor activities for kids – skiing, windsurfing, bike riding, hiking, climbing, skating or swimming. The more activities children try, the more encouraged they will be to expand their repertoire of skills. They'll also begin to view exercise as something associated with leisure and fun, rather than just a boring PE class at school.

• Invest in a pedometer for every family member (a very cheap item that measures the number of footsteps you take in a day). Set every child a target (10,000 for a teenager, less for younger kids) and make it into a bit of a competition, where you all compare figures at the end of the day. It's one way to spark children into moving a little more – and you can even supply a prize for the winner at the end of every week. While it may be a short-lived novelty for some families, kids will start to see the impact that even a little exercise can have on their stamina, energy levels and overall fitness. Once habits are established, however, there's a better chance that they'll continue.

• Don't underestimate the effect of housework on fitness. Many kids today are used to doing zilch around the house – which also prepares them in no way for adulthood. Even small children are capable of pushing a vacuum cleaner around (if erratically), carrying laundry from room to room, tidying away toys, washing dishes and setting the table. Although this doesn't sound like much exercise in itself, every little bit helps in the long run, and it does mean that your children aren't just 'sitting'. It's the sedentary part of children's lifestyles that seems to be causing the greatest problem with fitness and weight. Did you know, for example, that a child sitting in front of the television burns approximately 33 calories an hour, whereas a child standing burns 66 calories an hour? It's easy to see how even minor adjustments can affect weight loss and weight maintenance. OK, so few kids are likely to consider housework 'fun', but if their pocket money depends upon it, they are more likely to acquiesce. But remember, kids do enjoy responsibility, particularly when it is acknowledged and respected. If they are genuinely helping you, and you show enthusiasm and gratitude for their efforts, they will develop self-respect and take pride in their achievements. And everyone mucking in together for 20 minutes after school – as part of a normal routine – *can* actually be fun.

Inspiring lazy children

Have you got a non-starter on your hands? Some children seem to be much happier in front of a screen, or in a corner somewhere with a book. While these activities have their place in normal family life, chances are your child will not be getting the exercise he needs. Consider some of the following ideas:

• Put up a star chart for exercise. For every half-hour of activity, offer a star. A completed chart can be rewarded with anything your children fancy (within reason!) – a new football, a new tennis racquet or trainers, judo or skating lessons, a new book or video, or even just 30 minutes of playtime with you, doing whatever they want!

• Be sneaky. Park as far away as you can from the shops so that you'll have to walk further to get there. Send your child on local errands, or up and down the stairs to fetch things. Encourage them to make their own beds and to carry the shopping. All of these regular activities add up in terms of fitness.

• Talk to your child and try to work out why he doesn't like getting involved in sports or just running around in the park. It may be that he's had a bad experience in the playground, or he may feel that he's hopeless at sports. Talk things through and try to assess how you can help. Offer special coaching in a sport that many of his friends play. Encourage him to choose two or three sports that he's always wanted to try. You may find that his passion will be archery or dry-slope skiing, things that are not always routinely offered.

• Praise, praise, praise. If you offer lots of encouragement, your child will feel good about herself and take some pride in her achievements. Never put your child down or suggest that she isn't any good at a sport or other activity. Children learn confidence when they are encouraged, and they learn to like themselves when they feel that you approve of them.

• Don't nag or focus too much on the health benefits of exercising. While all children need to be educated about their bodies and their health needs, they don't want to feel that they are being lectured, or that they are under pressure to please you.

• In a 1999 survey, more than 1,200 children aged between 11 and 16 were asked about their attitude towards health and fitness. The youngsters said they wanted more information on how to be healthy – but they did not want to be lectured by adults. Take this advice to heart and offer some choices. Present information in a casual way – you'll open the door for discussion and an exchange of facts. Assess your own lifestyle and point out that you are concerned about how inactive you are. Ask your child's advice about becoming fitter and how the whole family can get more exercise. Make the information relevant. If you child is academic rather than sporty, point out that exercise can improve memory and concentration and reduce stress. If you have an 'armchair athlete', explain that all top stars (football, basketball, hockey, rugby, athletics, or whatever) need to train and practise hard. Offer to set up a training scheme that will improve your child's performance.

- Get involved. If you are out there kicking or batting a ball, they'll be much more likely to want to take part. Make fitness a family goal, with everyone playing a role.

- Offer appropriate choices to empower your child. Say, for example, what would you like to do today: play football in the park, go for a walk in the country, visit the local pool or take a trip to an adventure playground? Make sure all the options include some activity. Children like to feel that they are in control of their lives, and will believe that they have some stake in things when they are given choices.

- Cycling is a cheap and effective way to have an aerobic workout – and virtually all kids enjoy it. Younger children can cycle in their local park, while older kids can try longer rides. Cycling is also a great way to explore your local area. Contact your local council for information on cycling routes near you.

- Alternatively, kicking a football around, playing Frisbee or even a game of basketball seem like fun to most children and not too much like 'exercise'. Call up a few other parents and before you know it you will have a team. This will not only add to the competitive spirit but will provide a good opportunity for your children to interact with their peers – much better than having a one-to-one relationship with the TV!

Little couch potatoes

Studies show that even toddlers are now spending inordinate amounts of time in front of the television, and many of them even have television in their bedrooms. This is a crucial age for weight gain, and it is also an important stage at which to establish healthy habits. It's much harder to encourage activity in a child who has never spent much time outdoors or done any real form of exercise, and this is undoubtedly contributing to the problem of obesity in today's kids.

Most young children will be naturally active and it is important to encourage this instinctive behaviour from the very earliest days. Some children may need to be kept in a pushchair or on reins near busy streets, but always offer the opportunity to get out and walk or run. Keeping a child in one place for any length of time will curtail their natural enthusiasm and curiosity. It can be a trying task to keep a toddler safe in a busy city or even within a house, but it's fairly easy to child-proof your home for the few years that it matters, and it's even easier to take your child out to the park, the local tumble tots, adventure playground, swimming pool or even music and movement classes.

Here are some ideas to keep little ones active:

• Turn on the music and dance. Most children naturally respond to music and if you become involved, they'll think it's great fun.

• Set up a play gym in the sitting room, using cushions from chairs or a sofa.

• Invest in a baby bouncer, which will allow older babies to sit upright and use their legs to jump up and down.

• Fill a plastic pool or the bath with a little warm water and lots of toys. You'll create the ideal setting for 'splashaerobics'.

• If you've got a reluctant crawler or walker, set their favourite toys just out of reach. They'll soon learn that they have to move to get what they want. Make it into a game and have your little one chase the toy around a suitably safe room.

- Make sure your child has toys that encourage him to walk, push or pull. All of these activities invite action and improve coordination. He'll also learn a great deal about his world by experimenting.

- Invite round children of a similar age. Very few children will want to sit on their own if there is a group activity underway.

- Encourage older children to help around the house – carrying laundry to the washing machine, pushing a broom around the kitchen, or even helping to carry the shopping in from the car.

- Blow up a balloon and play volleyball, or just try to keep it in the air!

Quiet times are also important, but don't be tempted to use the video as a baby-sitter. Although every parent needs some peace and time to themselves, too much time in front of a television screen at an early age can encourage inactivity and make your child less enthusiastic about active pursuits.

Adolescent apathy

The teenage years are notorious for languorous living. However, this is understandable to a certain extent as many teenagers require more sleep than children who have not quite reached adolescence, as they grow and develop a great deal during these years. Not surprisingly, many adolescents have little energy or inclination to become involved in sporting activities, particularly if they're considered to be 'uncool'. Family outings may not hold the same appeal that they did when your adolescent was younger, and you'll need to find ways to keep him enthusiastic and, most importantly, fit.

It's crucially important to create and maintain relationships as your child grows up. If your child views you as the enemy, your advice is likely to be ignored to the point of rebellion. Obviously if sport or physical activity played a big part in her younger years, she's likely to continue to enjoy exercise. That's one of the reasons why it is so important to create healthy habits early on. However, if you are con-

TIPS FOR LAZY PARENTS

There's no question that many of us would prefer to unwind on our own terms, and after a busy day at the office, or with the children, the idea of exercise can be daunting. It's important therefore to focus on the fun element, and to choose activities that you will enjoy, too. For example, a family game in the park on a lazy Sunday might seem less appealing than a comfortable slouch in front of the television or in the garden, but everyone will benefit, and you'll have the opportunity to spend some real quality time with your kids. Take breaks to read the Sunday papers, or take a picnic and a book to make it into a whole day out. Consider visits to the gym, where children can attend their own activities while you do something that appeals to you. The hardest part of any type of exercise is getting out of the house. However, once you've started, you will almost certainly enjoy it, and you'll feel better afterwards.

If you have to force yourself to get out, do it. Try to hold in your mind the feelings of rejuvenation that follow a good long walk, work-out or even fun day out with the kids. Don't hesitate to offer trade-offs. Make it clear to your children that you will spend an hour or two doing exactly what they want to do, if you get the same deal in return. So, for example, you could schedule your Sunday to have a long walk or a game in the park with the kids, followed by a quiet period where you will be left in peace to read the paper, make some telephone calls or even take a nap. Similarly, you can offer trade-offs after school. You can agree to a half an hour or so in the park or at the local pool if your children will help to put away the food shopping later, help with dinner or even just promise to do their homework without a fuss.

Above all, try to be enthusiastic if you have active children. If they sense that you are bored or less than happy being involved, it will ruin their pleasure and they'll start to make negative associations with the activity in question. They'll also think it is normal for adults to dislike exercise, which gives them the idea that it's not all that important. If you can't fit it into a busy day, ask an older neighbourhood child to play with them, or call on aunts and uncles and even grandparents to play a role.

cerned about activity levels now, having either neglected that side of family life to some extent, or been unable to persuade your child to become involved in any sports or activities, it's not too late to make some changes.

The advantage of dealing with older children is that they can understand and reason (well, perhaps only on a good day!). You can best make headway by making things relevant to their daily life. Once again, draw parallels between famous sportspeople, dancers, athletes or even scientists, if that's appropriate. Everyone, in every walk of life, can benefit from exercise and you need to find a way to get that message through. Whether it's the reduction in stress, or the increase in brain power and endurance that your teenager will respond to, there will be a way to convince them that exercise can help them do better at something they're interested in. Whatever you do, try not to lecture or nag. Offer positive choices and let your teenager make her own decisions. Just ensure that the choices you offer are realistic and active!

Adolescence is a stressful period, and many teenagers find the transition from childhood to adulthood very difficult. You may lock horns on many occasions throughout these years but, just like small children, adolescents do need to be guided and they need praise and encouragement. If your child feels good about herself throughout these years, she is more likely to communicate with you, with her peers and with other adults. She'll also have more respect for herself and her body. If a teenager takes pride in her body and her achievements, she'll be more likely to make healthy decisions. Raising self-esteem can be crucial to your child's long-term success in any part of her life.

It's well known that children who are involved in sports and even music have less free time to experiment with drugs and alcohol, so focus on keeping your teenager active from the earliest possible moment. Busy, motivated teenagers have little free time for leisure activities that can harm their health.

Here are some ideas to help get your teenager moving:

• The star system may be a little out of date for a teenager, but the principle remains the same. Offer rewards – and plenty of them – for behaviour that you want to encourage. For example, if your child agrees to attend a sport of his choice once or twice a week, you could offer a lift (and possibly a ticket) to the cinema at the weekend, or a new CD.

- Dancing is a good aerobic sport. Many unathletic children are very keen on music. Indulge this passion and maybe club together with a few other parents to get a karaoke machine and some CDs that you can swap. Make sure your child has a room where she can feel free to move about comfortably, away from the eyes of her siblings or parents. She'll be much more likely to move around if she's not being watched! You can also give it a try yourself – if you're not worried about how badly you dance or sing it'll encourage them to feel the same and do it simply for the enjoyment it gives.

- Set a series of fitness assessments, and offer a reward if your teenager can produce some good results and improvement over a period of time. Ask her to set up the programme (including sit-ups, running around the block or a track, running up stairs) and offer to time her.

- Keep up the family activities. Many older children find it embarrassing to be seen with their parents, but agree, as a family, to at least one session together a week. Try to make sure these times involve some physical activity. Similarly, family holidays are still appropriate for teenagers, and you can choose one that will appeal to the whole family – with sports and games for all ages.

- Encourage your child to get a part-time job helping out at the local swimming pool, sports club, football club or gym. She will be more likely to be inspired if she's in an environment that encourages fitness. The long summer holidays can be spent helping out at local school or sports club activity weeks, where older children and teenagers are involved in teaching and training the younger children. The majority of teenagers will respond to some responsibility, and will probably want to impress the younger children with their knowledge and skill.

- Consider some of the summer camp or adventure holidays set up for teenagers. It may be beyond your budget, but many offer concessions, particularly if your child can be of some assistance. Similarly, a summer job acting as a supervisor will keep her active, and she'll probably learn new sports and skills that can become passions.

- Most teenagers will respond to some competition. Set up a regular game of tennis or squash together. It's one way to ensure that you stay fit, and you might find that you are soon out of your depth!

- Offer to arrange courses in some of the more varied sports on offer – horseback riding, mountain biking, athletics, diving, archery, martial arts, indoor climbing, or skiing. Anything that moves muscles will, in the long run, work towards fitness goals.

Setting goals

One way to motivate all family members is to set regular goals and work towards achieving them. Every child and adult may have their own reasons for becoming fitter – to make a team at school, to lose some weight on their tummy or legs, to have more energy or simply to lose a little weight overall and feel healthier. Talk to your kids – at the dinner table is ideal – about what their goals might be and encourage them to establish a realistic goal for fitness.

Set small challenges and let them see the results. For example, running is a great way to show how quickly we can get fit when we try. Get every family member to run around the block and time themselves. Carry on for a week or so, and they will soon see that their time improves dramatically. Then make it twice around the block, and then three times. Even kids can't fail to be amazed by how much their stamina and speed improves with just a little effort, and you may well encourage a regular habit of jogging. The same goes for swimming or just about any other sport. Get them to set goals for what they want to achieve (mastering a David Beckham-style curling free kick, for example, or getting to the top at a climbing wall, a belt in a martial art, a badge in swimming lessons, or making the 'A' team – or any team – at school) and encourage them to work at it until they succeed. Every little success breeds more enthusiasm.

Special notes for very overweight kids

If your child is very overweight or feels uncomfortable about his size for any reason, exercise can be an embarrassing and daunting experience. All of the above ideas may sound hopelessly idealistic if you have a child who is genuinely upset by the idea of exercising, losing face, or opening themselves up to ridicule. It's important to be hugely sensitive to your child's feelings, and to empathize with their position. Forcing them into activities that they hate will only undermine their confidence, and putting themselves in the position of being teased by other children will defeat the purpose.

However, the bottom line is that all kids – and overweight kids in particular – need to learn to exercise regularly. And there are things that you can do to make it easier for them to achieve an acceptable level of fitness.

- First of all, make sure your child is appropriately dressed for any activity. Squeezing them into a football kit, aerobics leotard, ballet tights or any sports clothing that is too small will exacerbate the problem. Ensure that your child has clothing that fits and that hides any part of his body that make him feel self-conscious – however, it shouldn't envelop him like a tent and make him stand out. If children look the part, they are much more likely to feel involved and, if they are comfortable, they will not feel that they stand out from the crowd.

- Consideration also needs to be given to your child's personal needs and feelings. A 2001 study found that fun, success, variety, freedom, family participation, peer support and enthusiastic leadership encourage and maintain participation: conversely, failure, embarrassment, competition, boredom, regimentation and injuries discourage further participation. So get it right. Ensure your child is involved in activities she enjoys, and where there are other children who are not stick thin.

- Children who are physically self-conscious, or who feel different from their peers, may feel uncomfortable about participating in team activities. Fear of failure or public embarrassment – as well as fear of letting their parents down – can also make some children reluctant to play team sports. Some children, like many adults, may just not be interested in team sports, but they can still maintain an excellent level of fitness by engaging in other activities that don't emphasize competition. As long as your child does not become sedentary, there's no need to worry if he resists joining organized sports activities.

- One of the major problems with encouraging overweight children to become fitter is an actual fear of vigorous exercise. If they are out of breath after climbing a flight of stairs, they will be daunted by the prospect of anything more demanding. Start small. Begin by walking together as a family, for example, or use a pedometer to increase the number of steps he takes in any given day. Make sure that your child has developed a reasonable level of basic fitness before involving him in an activity where the other children are likely to be fitter.

- Encourage your child to take up a lifelong activity, such as cycling, running, martial arts, or hiking. These activities promote fitness on an individual, not competitive level. You could also suggest wrestling, tennis, swimming, or gymnastics teams. In these activities, the sport is individual or one-on-one, but participants can still earn team points. Also, the pressure is not so dramatic when there is failure.

- Children know if they are overweight and don't need to be reminded or singled out. They need acceptance, encouragement and love.

- Remember that they will be embarrassed if they are forced into situations where they are not comfortable. An overweight child is not going to feel good about getting into a bathing suit if she is surrounded by slimmer peers, and it may well ruin the whole experience of swimming for her. Choose activities where their weight will not be highlighted.

CASE HISTORY: Eleanor

Eleanor had been overweight from a young age, and had always been embarrassed in any exercise situation – particularly at school, where she had a gym kit that looked ridiculous on her, and also because she could never keep up. As a result she was often taunted and no-one ever wanted her in their group or team. She began to make excuses in order to miss PE and games, and her teachers eventually gave up trying to motivate her. The same thing occurred in her home life – she stopped hanging around with friends who liked to cycle or go swimming together, and she became lonely.

When she was 12, she realized that her weight was becoming a real problem and asked her parents for help. She was taken to her doctor, who explained the importance of exercise and suggested a 'fat camp' club at the local health centre. At the outset, she was aghast at the idea that she had to resort to exercising with 'fat kids', but she grudgingly agreed. It was a revelation. Not only was she not the fattest in the group by far (something to which she had been accustomed), but she was also given exercises that were appropriate to her fitness levels, so she didn't feel like a failure. What's more, the other kids also struggled to get fit, so she didn't stand out in any way. Taunting and teasing played no part in the proceedings – in fact, the staff and the children themselves were very supportive. Eleanor soon began to enjoy the visits and, over the next year, managed to lose a little weight while growing more than 15 cm (6 in) in height, which had a dramatic effect on her appearance. Mastering the fitness routines gave her more confidence to try other sports, and she was soon fit enough to take part in an after-school badminton club that she wanted to try.

To her great surprise, too, she performed well on sports day, which made her feel great. Eleanor now enjoys exercise and spends more time with fitter friends – as well as those she made at the fat club, which she still attends regularly.

• Consider enrolling your child in a class with other overweight kids. Although it's important not to label kids as overweight, categorize them or make them feel that they can only exercise when there are other heavy children around, it can help them to start an exercise programme when they are in the company of kids who share the same problems. In some ways, this type of activity acts a bit like group therapy – kids can be themselves and be honest about their weight problems with others who are in the same boat. In addition, the exercises will have been developed with the problems associated with overweight – stamina, energy, flexibility, embarrassment and so on – in mind. If your child is very overweight and concerned about it, he may well feel much happier being with kids who are experiencing the same problems. Don't force it, but offer it as an option.

• Pay close attention to every success. It's never a good idea to have weight loss as a goal. As I outlined earlier, the best way to deal with overweight kids is to stabilize weight so that they grow into it. Giving them unachievable targets may be dispiriting and cause them to lose interest. It's better to work on small goals and little successes – an increase in the number of laps they can swim, the extra 10 minutes of cycling they achieve, the increased number of sit-ups or minutes on an exercise bike, better skills at basketball – even their new-found ability to touch their toes. Make every success a celebration. Weight loss will undoubtedly be the result of a good exercise programme, but that should be an additional 'bonus', even if it does serve to motivate your child more.

• Don't force your child into exercises with other kids if she is not ready. Anything that gets her up and moving is enough to begin with – such as brownies, cub scouts, craft classes or horseback riding. This will make them more active and more likely to try other things. Start small and expand her interests when she shows enthusiasm.

• Talk to your child about feelings of embarrassment, and try to instil some self-pride and self-liking in your child. I'll go into this in more detail in the following chapter, but, for now, recognize that he may have emotional issues about his weight, and very real fears about what other people think of him, and how they'll react. Acknowledge these fears and work with your child to overcome them. Help him to increase his stamina by giving him small projects or goals at which he can succeed. Teach him, for instance, that red faces are common in lots of healthy, fit people of normal weight. If he's embarrassed by sweating, buy him a suitable deodorant and clothing that is less likely to draw attention to the problem. Explain that feeling clumsy is normal when we are unfit, and that coordination improves over time. Whatever you do, don't dismiss his concerns out of hand. They are very real to him, and may be the reason why he has given up on active pursuits in the first place.

• Many overweight children lack willpower because they have such a poor self-image. 'What's the point …' is a common complaint amongst kids struggling with their weight. People who feel good about themselves are that much more likely to look after their bodies: the opposite also holds true. It doesn't mean your child is lazy or slovenly; he's just lost the enthusiasm for taking care of himself. Encourage him all the way – again, celebrating every success, no matter how small. Encourage him to continue, even when he feels like giving up, by explaining how exercise can make him feel better on all levels.

There's no doubt that a little regular exercise will eventually improve your child's moods and emotional health and, once you get the ball rolling, these effects will help to promote a greater interest and longer staying power. Studies of adolescents have shown that 20 minutes of aerobic activity three times per week has significant positive effects on their health, and can help control depression and anxiety. Children involved in fitness-related activities have a stronger self-image, along with more self-confidence, and they demonstrate greater improvement in their skill at sport and health-related fitness.

Leisure activities

Making the transition to exercising regularly does mean a change in leisure activities. Kids are used to sitting in front of the TV, games console, computer or even a book, and changing their habits is one of the most important things you can do to encourage healthier lifestyle habits. These changes may not be popular at the outset, but stick to your guns. New rules, new routines and a new regime are necessary in order to get the whole family fitter and healthier. I can tell you right now that all kids will resist, and you may be tempted to give in before you have even established the ground rules. But one of the most important jobs we as parents can do is to help our children establish habits that will contribute to their health both now and in the future. Discipline and rules are essential if we are to teach our children anything. Remember, you are in charge and you can ultimately make the decisions. Parenting is not an easy job, but it's necessary to be tough sometimes.

Establishing, monitoring and modelling good habits is important in all facets of life. Setting the standard for your children by establishing the rules of your home and modelling a healthful lifestyle is a first step in guiding your children towards pursuing lifelong healthy practices. Hence it is the responsibility of parents and care providers to establish, monitor and model good habits concerning the use of media. The following recommendations may help:

Preventing the TV or computer from ruling the roost

- Limit television viewing to no more than one to two hours per day. If your child plays on a games console or the computer as well, this figure should cover total screen time. I suggest an hour a day for all of these types of activities during the week, extending it to two or three hours a day on weekends. But no session should be longer than half an hour (unless there is a good programme on television that lasts longer). Children can choose how they divide up their viewing/playing time. For example, they may choose no TV one night, and instead spend an hour on the playstation, or opt for half an hour of each. In our household, the games console is out of bounds during the school week. This rule was put in place when it was first purchased and therefore never really questioned, although from time to time there are pleas for exceptions – which are considered, too. On the weekends, as long as homework is done, virtually anything goes – but the rule of thumb is that for every hour on the playstation, there has to be at least another hour of exercise or playing outside. On many weekends, they don't play on the playstation at all – choosing instead to be outside with their friends or playing sports.

- This type of rule does mean knowing how much TV your children watch, and not hesitating to reduce the time. Many kids have TVs in their bedrooms, or games consoles/computers, and parents really don't have any idea of how much time is spent on them. Check constantly – it's the only way to keep tabs.

- Plan television viewing in advance. Use a TV guide or newspaper to select the shows your family wants to watch. Too often we get into the habit of flicking through channels and watching for the sake of watching. Encourage them to make choices. If their time is limited, they'll be much more likely to do so.

- Be a good role model. Though television may seem benign, our own habits and attitudes in front of the screen influence our children's health. According to a recent study, the more television you watch, the more your child watches. If we are watching TV, we are also limiting important time that could be spent talking with each other and sharing in each other's lives.

- Minimize the influence of television in your home. To keep the TV from being a central part of the home:

  1 Keep the TV off during family mealtimes
  2 Make conversation the priority in your home
  3 Don't centre furniture around the TV
  4 Try not to allow TVs in individual bedrooms as this isolates family members, reduces family interaction and increases the amount of TV watched.

- Avoid allowing children under the age of two to watch television. Research on early brain development shows that for healthy brain growth, as well as development of appropriate social, emotional and cognitive skills, children of this age have a critical need for direct interactions with parents and care-givers. Plus, if a child has never learned to use TV as entertainment at a young age, he'll develop other interests early on, including reading or looking at story books, drawing, or just talking.

• Don't use television, video games, or recreational computer time as a reward. According to research by the Nemours Foundation in the US, using these media as rewards may make their use seem more important to children.

• Provide alternatives to television, video games and recreational computer use. Parents and care providers are responsible for how much time their children spend in front of the TV, computer, or video screen. Encourage both indoor and outdoor activities for your children – particularly those that encourage active play. Parents often give in to the litany of complaints – 'I'm bored', 'There's nothing to do' – and allow more TV or games than they should. You can preclude this by sitting down with your children and coming up with 100 different things that can be done when they are bored or when it's raining. Stick it on the fridge and point it out when they complain.

Teaching time management

Limiting time with various media will teach your children how to plan their time, and this will make it much easier to fit in other activities, such as exercise. One of the greatest skills that any adult can learn is time management, because it helps not only to ensure that activities are prioritized, but also that time is used most effectively, allowing space for essential leisure, relaxation and fun. Because children's schedules are now almost as fast-paced and packed as most adults, it's a skill that children will undoubtedly benefit from learning, and one that will stand them in good stead in the future.

If your children are young, you'll need to be heavily involved in the process, perhaps planning out their time and schedule for them, with their input. Planning a schedule also offers a good opportunity to discuss activities and priorities – the importance of exercise and 'down' time that doesn't involve being in front of the TV. And you can use this to uncover areas where your child is most stressed, overworked or undertaking activities that he either no longer enjoys or that subject him to too much pressure.

Older children and adolescents should be encouraged regularly to manage their time by developing schedules and by listing their preferences and priorities. The same system can be applied to children of all ages, but it's important that you are involved at some stage, if only to gauge changes in your child's interests or to uncover areas of potential stress.

Setting priorities

Sit down with your child and think about priorities. The obvious ones are exercise, sleep, eating together, 'talking' time, school, homework, free time, time with friends, and family activities. List all of her current activities then get her to add any activities that she enjoys enormously and which aren't on the list. You might be surprised by what she says! Now get her to rate the entries on the list according to their importance to her and how much enjoyment she gets from them. Use this as a talking point. If you feel some activities that she wants to drop are worthwhile, explain why and be prepared for concessions on both sides. The aim here is to reduce over-scheduling, and make it possible to set up a routine that allows all of the important aspects of life to be fitted in easily.

This may all sound like hard work, but remember that despite being largely sedentary, today's children often have very busy schedules with no real time to relax or recharge their batteries. This contributes to the problem of stress in children, which in turn impacts on weight. Furthermore, a child whose schedule is too tightly orchestrated will be exhausted and less likely to want to take part in active pursuits. What you want to achieve are plenty of 'free time' slots, where kids can do their own thing away from the TV or computer. They are much more likely to go out and kick a ball with some friends if there is time in the schedule to do what they like, or they can choose to go swimming or to the park or anything else that keeps them relaxed, happy and active. And pastimes like reading a book shouldn't be discouraged – as long as they're active at other times. Relaxation is an important part of a balanced lifestyle, and as long as it doesn't take place in front of the TV, it should be encouraged. Relaxed children tend to be much more able to cope with the pressures of modern life, and have a more balanced approach to it.

Planning a schedule

The purpose of a schedule is to set a routine, and it will help to encourage your child to get on with the job at hand, particularly if he knows that some 'fun' activities are planned as well. Make sure there is a good balance between play, fun and work, and that you leave completely free periods. Make sure your child is involved in the process. Ask him to have a go at scheduling his activities before you begin, then work with him to fine tune it.

Some children's days might be very busy, in which case you need to offer short breaks more often. Choose a day or days when they have friends round, and try to keep at least one day a week free from homework to allow for complete relaxation and a free choice of activities. Slot in an hour or so every day for exercise or sport, at least an hour of 'free time' (in which children can play; most are active when they play), and, of course, the all-essential (to kids) media viewing slot. Allow time for homework, but also 'family' time, which is crucially important to the family dynamic and the emotional health of all family members.

Try to find a good balance between 'being' and 'doing'. With better time management, both you and your children can be more productive, experience improved relationships and enjoy more good times with the minimum of stress and anxiety. And the most important thing is that it will become clear that the 'too busy' excuse – for exercise, homework or anything else – is no longer relevant. Kids who learn to plan their time will benefit in later years – when they have exams, busy jobs and families. They'll have learned to prioritize the important things such as exercise, leisure activities they enjoy, time with family and friends, and simply 'down time'. And they'll also see that not wasting hours in front of the television frees them up to do more interesting things.

Time management doesn't have to be done every week – in fact, after a couple of weeks, you'll find that your kids have established a healthy routine and manage to fit much more in, as well as having more time for leisure. And that's a much healthier way to live.

What about sleep?

Although this chapter deals mainly with exercise and leisure – getting kids up and active, and away from the telly – it is important to touch upon the other side of the equation – sleep. In the introduction to this book, we learned that one of the side-effects of obesity is poor or disrupted sleep, as well as a condition called 'sleep apnoea', a serious and debilitating sleep disorder.

Sleep apnoea is characterized by brief but numerous involuntary breathing pauses during sleep. These breathing pauses cause awakenings throughout the night, making it impossible for sleep apnoea sufferers to enjoy a night of deep, restorative sleep. People with sleep apnoea often feel sleepy during the day and their concentration and daytime performance suffer.

The repercussions of sleep apnoea and poor sleep for children are vast. When children do not get the sleep they need, their health and performance suffers, and difficulties in school are an all-too-common result. However, sleep deprivation in children is often overlooked or attributed to attention-deficit or behaviour disorders.

How much sleep does your child need?

Sleep needs differ dramatically between children, just as they do between adults. However, there is no excuse for thinking that a child can get by on what an adult gets. Sleep is crucially important in childhood and adolescence, and there are very, very few children who do not need to get at least the average required hours. The table opposite lists the average number of hours that each age group requires. Don't be surprised if your child doesn't fit the norm exactly. It's simply helpful to have an idea of what to expect – and what to aim for. If you find your child is getting dramatically less or more than required, you may need to assess why.

Not only does obesity contribute to sleep problems, but sleep problems can also contribute to obesity. A 1999 study found that building up a sleep 'debt' over a matter of days can impair metabolism and disrupt hormone levels. After restricting 11 healthy young adults

AGE	NUMBER OF HOURS	NUMBER OF SLEEP PERIODS/SPECIAL NOTES
Newborns	16 to 18	In periods throughout the day – about half will be during the night and half during the day
3 to 6 months	15	Sleep occurs over about four or five periods, with about two-thirds occurring at night. Somewhere between three and six months a baby will normally begin to sleep for long stretches at night
6 to 12 months	14 to 15	Daytime sleep during this period is normally reduced from about 4 to $2\frac{1}{2}$ hours, which means that night-time sleeping is increased accordingly. Naps will probably be regular (two a day, for example)
1 to 2 years	14	Naps still make up between 1 and $2\frac{1}{2}$ hours of sleep, with the remainder taking place at night. Most children drop the morning nap by the age of about two. Healthy two-year-olds are capable of sleeping for about 12 hours at night without waking
3 to 6 years	11 to 13 hours	The afternoon nap normally disappears around age three or four, although some sleepier children may benefit from a rest in the afternoons
7 to 9 years	9 to 11 hours	Children may take longer to fall asleep, and this figure does not take into consideration the time between lights out and falling asleep. These hours should be good-quality sleep only
10 to 11 years	8 to 11 hours	Children of this age often don't get what is required, and many parents are surprised by how much children do need in these pre-pubescent years
11 to 18 years	9.5 hours plus	Adolescents do need more sleep than younger children approaching their teenage years and, according to research, very few get more than about 6 hours a night

to four hours' sleep for six nights, researchers found their ability to process glucose (sugar) in the blood had declined – in some cases to the level of diabetics. This, understandably, has significant long-term consequences for weight control.

Recent research has also found that sleep deprivation may increase appetite. Because the psychological manifestations of fatigue, sleep and hunger are similar, we sometimes confuse them and eat not when we're hungry but when we're sleepy.

When children are not well rested, they'll obviously be less inclined to exercise. Additionally, when deprived of adequate sleep, there is a strong tendency to exercise at a reduced intensity. Hence, a rested person may walk two miles in 30 minutes, while the poorly rested person is likely to go at half that speed, cover half the distance and burn half the calories in the same amount of time.

Lack of sleep can also affect metabolism due to its effects on hormone levels. In particular, sleep loss affects the body's levels of hormones such as cortisone, insulin and growth hormone. Cortisone (the stress hormone) also increases in response to emotional or physical stress, and lack of sleep is considered one of these 'stresses'. Cortisone then raises insulin levels, which then promote fat storage and inhibit fat loss. When levels of growth hormones drop as a result of inadequate sleep, fat storage and a loss of muscle mass are the result.

And if all that isn't enough, it has been shown that when most people are deprived of sleep they tend to consume more calories than they require to maintain their body weight. Some studies have also indicated that a tired person tends to crave sweet, high-carbohydrate foods. Combine this with elevated cortisone and insulin, and the balance is set in favour of fat storage. What can you do?

Ensuring a good night's sleep

• Turn off the TV at least an hour before bedtime, so that your
  child isn't too stimulated to sleep. The same goes for games
  consoles and computers. These also tend to push bedtimes later
  and later while the kids 'finish a battle' or a 'match'. Don't even
  put yourself in the position of having to allow a later bedtime
  because of these excuses.

- Keep up with exercise – physically tired children are much more likely to sleep than those who have been inactive all day long.

- Set in place a good sleep routine. For younger children that means starting about 30–60 minutes in advance of bedtime, and including a warm bath, a story, a chat and a wind-down period. Older children will also benefit from a strong routine – a bath, and time to read quietly in their rooms before switching off the lights.

- Remember that tired children do not behave like exhausted adults – they may appear hyperactive, fidgety and bursting with energy. The key is to get them to bed a long time before these types of symptoms set in, otherwise they'll be too wound up to sleep. Some people have found that putting kids to bed 30 minutes earlier can make the all the difference for children who find it hard to settle.

- Exercise should be avoided in the 60–90 minutes before bedtime, as it can prevent children from falling asleep.

- Do not allow caffeine and sugary snacks wherever possible, as these can inhibit both falling asleep and staying asleep. A glass of milk, or a slice of turkey, cheese or wholemeal toast before they clean their teeth is fine. Kids with blood sugar problems will also sleep better if their blood sugar levels don't dip too low in the night.

- Instil in your children an understanding of why sleep is important – for concentrating, energy, balanced moods, learning and even weight control.

- Be firm. It is a parent's responsibility to set rules that will ensure good health for their children. Don't give in to demands that will affect your child's well-being. Set rules and stick to them. And when you say no, mean it.

In the Resources section you will find a number of organizations that offer advice on sleep difficulties (see page 258).

Creating a balanced lifestyle with plenty of time for fresh air, exercise, healthy leisure activities and sleep is crucial for all children, and particularly so for those who are experiencing problems with their weight. But creating a better lifestyle also has the added benefit of freeing up time for family and interaction between family members, something that is often sorely neglected in today's busy society. The impact of this can be crucial for you child's emotional health. And given that so many problems associated with obesity come down to your child's emotions, his self-respect and self-esteem, it is an area that needs attention in all families. In the next chapter we'll examine the importance of emotional health, and how you can achieve a balanced family life in which all members thrive.

Chapter Six

Building a Healthy Self-Image

Being overweight is a bit of a double-edged sword when it comes to emotional health. Not only are children with lower self-esteem or emotional issues more likely to suffer from overweight, but the self-esteem and self-respect of even the emotionally healthiest children can take a huge battering when they have a weight problem. Not surprisingly, this compounds the problem and increases the likelihood of even more weight gain.

In Chapter 2 we touched on how self-esteem and emotional health can be an important influence on a child's weight. Furthermore, we learned that an unhealthy relationship with food – where it becomes a source of comfort and a way of alleviating boredom, stress, anxiety, depression and unhappiness – is one of the biggest problems that many overweight children have. But what can parents do to tip the balance? How can you make an unhappy, overweight child blossom again, so that he will take an interest in active leisure pursuits, sustain healthy friendships and feel good about himself? No depressed or bullied child is miraculously going to find the impetus to make changes towards a healthier weight – they simply won't have the motivation to look after themselves, their bodies, their health and their appearance, if they have a poor self-image.

In this chapter we'll look at how to turn the tables in order to help your child build a healthy self-image and feel good about themselves. We'll examine how you can encourage self-esteem and self-respect, as well as an interest in weight – without denting your child's confidence. Changing the family dynamic is one important way of doing this. Many overweight children feel isolated and unable to share their problems. By creating a supportive and loving unit, where everyone is valued, overweight children can come to terms with their problem, and, as part of a family, seek solutions that will make them feel better about themselves and more able to cope with the normal pressures of growing up.

To begin with, let's look at the issues that overweight children face, often on a day-to-day basis:

• Overweight children tend to suffer more from anxiety and have poorer social skills than normal-weight children. At one extreme, these problems may lead to misbehaving and disrupting the classroom; at the other, they may cause social withdrawal. Stress and anxiety also interfere with learning. School-related anxiety can create a vicious cycle in which ever-growing worry fuels ever-declining academic performance.

• Social isolation and low self-esteem create overwhelming feelings of hopelessness in some overweight children. When children lose hope that their lives will improve, they are well on the way to depression. A depressed child may lose interest in normal activities, sleep more than usual or cry a lot. Some depressed children hide their sadness and appear emotionally flat instead. Either way, depression is as serious in children as it is in adults.

• One study of more than 90,000 teenagers found that overweight kids are more likely to have smaller social networks than their non-overweight peers. Researchers found that overweight students were 70 per cent less likely than their healthy-weight counterparts to be listed as friends of their peers. Although the overweight students listed classmates as their friends, the 'friends' didn't reciprocate.

• Overweight adolescents are more likely than normal-weight children to be victims of bullying, or be bullies themselves, a Canadian study found, bolstering evidence that being fat endangers emotional as well as physical health. The study, which was published in *Paediatrics*, in 2002, found that obese girls were about twice as likely to be physically bullied, on a weekly basis, than normal-weight girls; among obese boys the risk was slightly lower but still substantially higher than for normal-weight boys. Obese girls were also more than five times more likely than normal-weight girls to physically bully other youngsters at least once weekly. Among boys the risk of being physically aggressive was only slightly increased, but they were more than twice as likely to make fun of others and spread lies and rumours than normal-weight boys. The researchers concluded that 'The social and psychological ramifications induced by the bullying-victimization process may hinder the social development of overweight and obese youth, because adolescents are extremely reliant on peers for social support, identity and self-esteem'.

- Child psychologist Sylvia Rimm, author of *Rescuing the Emotional Lives of Overweight Children*, says that many schools with anti-bullying programmes don't specifically address overweight youngsters. According to Rimm, reducing bullying could help youngsters overcome their weight problems. Bullying perpetuates those problems because it isolates them and, as she says, 'the only thing left for overweight kids is food and television'.

- In the UK, a 2003 study found that girls as young as nine are resorting to dieting after being teased about their weight. One in five nine-year-old girls and nearly as many boys had been bullied by classmates for being fat, the study found. Experts are concerned the taunts are contributing to the slimming fad among children, particularly young girls.

- As obesity increases and fitness decreases, children are developing chronic diseases at earlier ages. Overweight and obese children tend to grow quicker and are sometimes mistaken for older children. They are more likely to be discriminated against and to develop negative attitudes about being overweight, according to a 2003 study, which surveyed nearly 5,000 children. It found that 30 per cent of girls and nearly 25 per cent of boys were consistently teased by peers about their weight. And it's not much better at home, especially for girls – 28 per cent reported teasing by family members, while 16 per cent of the boys suffered in this way. Researchers say the fallout of such torment includes a higher than normal rate of low self-esteem, depression and suicidal thoughts.

• The longer a child is overweight, the more he or she is at risk of depression and other mental health disorders. Researchers have found that obesity carries a large social stigma and may bring on depression if it negatively affects self-esteem, body image or social mobility. It may even disrupt the normal hormonal pathways. And depression may also bring on obesity, if a child lacks the energy to exercise or is immobilized by stress.

• One fascinating study, published in the *Journal of the American Medical Association*, found that obese kids were 5.5 times more likely to have an impaired quality of life than healthy kids, putting their life experience on par with that of kids undergoing chemotherapy treatment for cancer. 'Obese children reported scores [on a quality of life survey] that were as bad as cancer patients in each and every domain of life,' says Dr Jeffrey Schwimmer, of the University of California in San Diego. 'We were surprised it was that bad.' The study also found that obese children missed an average of four days of school a month, compared to less than a day for kids of average weight.

• The extent and nature of teasing of overweight children has been illustrated by a number of UK studies. One found that 96 per cent of overweight adolescent girls reported hurtful and humiliating comments and derogatory names. There is also research suggesting that many health professionals, including doctors, dieticians and nurses, share 'anti-fat' prejudices. A study by Dr Andrew Hill of Leeds University found that 14 per cent of 12-year-olds and 18 per cent of nine-year-olds were regularly teased for being 'fat', yet around half of these children weren't medically obese or even overweight. 'All those teased, and some of the teasers showed lower self-esteem, were more likely to diet and more likely to dislike their bodies,' he said. 'We need to remember, when dealing with obesity, that psychological factors are very important and eating disorders such as anorexia are the flip side of the coin.'

• In one study, childhood obesity was associated with a 2.5 times greater likelihood of a disorder known as oppositional defiant disorder, defined as an ongoing pattern of uncooperative, defiant, hostile behaviour toward authority figures. The disorder is more common in boys, but the researchers found it to be elevated in both obese boys and girls. Childhood obesity specialist Dr Sarah Barlow says a child with defiance disorder is less likely to set limits for himself or follow those set by parents, and this could easily lead to obesity.

Whatever way you look at it, this does not make happy reading. Obviously some of these studies concentrate on children who have been obese for long periods of time and may be dangerously over-weight. But it's important to remember that in our society weight is a terribly emotive issue, and the intense focus on being thin can make overweight children not only unhappy and isolated, but also the butt of jokes and the target of bullying. Whether your child is in this position now is largely irrelevant. Unless you help her to do something about her weight, she could be. She may also be hiding her distress behind apathy or a brave face, and you may not be aware that a problem even exists. It all sounds rather dramatic, and perhaps unrelated to the average overweight child, but it's impor-tant to remember that self-esteem and self-image are very fragile as children are growing up, and they can be easily knocked – setting in place emotional problems that can affect children for the rest of their lives.

Another key thing to remember is the fact that children's weight problems may well be exacerbated by the difficulties they are expe-riencing. It's hard for any unhappy adult to drag themselves up and dust themselves off time after time, and a child may be tempted just to give up and find further solace in food and unhealthy eating. It takes a very strong and determined child to find the motivation to change their lifestyle and move in a more positive direction in the face of teasing, taunting, bullying and the corresponding negative self-image that they develop. There's no doubt about it – kids can be very unkind to one another and you do not, as a parent, want your child to be put into a position of being the target.

One way around this is to work on raising your child's self-esteem and self-respect, and improving his body image, so that he can withstand some of the abuse and cope with the negative feelings associated with overweight – as well as find the motivation required to change.

Encouraging a child with a weight problem

Before looking at how you can boost your child's self-esteem, let's examine how the various ways you can encourage an overweight child to adopt a healthier lifestyle. Because of their fragile self-esteem, it is important to go about this in the right way, so as not to exacerbate any emotional issues that might be contributing to the problem.

• First of all, it is important not to label a child as fat, chubby, plump or even 'big'. Children hold great store by what their parents tell them, and build their self-identities on what they hear about themselves. By labelling a child you can undermine her confidence and create a self-fulfilling prophecy.

• Overweight and obesity typically indicates poor self-esteem and a negative body image. Teasing or embarrassing your child, or pointing out a perceived problem repeatedly, will do nothing but encourage these problems.

• Encourage your child in what she does well; let her know that you love, value and approve of her.

• Make sure your child has attractive and fashionable clothes. For one thing it will help her to take pride in her appearance, which

IS OBESITY AN EATING DISORDER?

In some children, obesity may well be related to an eating disorder; in fact, an unhealthy relationship with food, fed by emotional problems that lead to erratic behaviour with food or in other areas of their life, would be classified as an eating disorder, although it may be less serious than disorders such as bulimia and anorexia. But it's worth noting that overweight children are at risk of these types of eating disorders. And studies show that children who are placed on diets and deprived of food are more likely to associate negative feelings with food and suffer from eating disorders later in life. Further research indicates that parents who try to police what their children eat overzealously may inadvertently create depression, shame, feelings of abandonment and anxiety – all of which can contribute to the threat of an eating disorder developing. One study found that binge eating and night-eating disorders account for as many as 10–20 per cent of people who seek treatment for obesity.

Some overweight children may have developed a binge-eating disorder as a result of their unhealthy relationship with food. Common symptoms include:

• Eating frequently and repeatedly
• Feeling out of control and unable to stop eating during binges
• Often eating rapidly and secretly, or may snack and nibble all day long
• Feeling guilty and ashamed of binge eating
• A history of diet failures
• A tendency towards depression or just feeling low
• Obesity.

People who have a binge-eating disorder do not regularly vomit, over-exercise, or abuse laxatives like bulimics do. They may be genetically predisposed to weigh more than the cultural ideal (which at present is exceedingly unrealistic), so they diet, make themselves hungry and then binge in response to that hunger. Or they may eat for emotional reasons: to comfort themselves, avoid threatening situations and numb emotional pain.

If this sounds like your child, you may need to get some additional help from a health expert. Your doctor can put you in touch with a consultant who can help.

can spark an interest in looking after herself. It's also important that overweight kids don't feel different from their peers, and that you avoid giving some of those nastier peers further grounds for teasing. Helping them to look good is one way of encouraging kids to feel good about themselves, which can help to shift unhealthy patterns. Some parents avoid buying their kids nice clothing when they are overweight on the premise that they will not be encouraged to lose weight – many adults hold by the same concept, buying clothes a size too small as motivation for weight loss. It won't work for kids. It will just make them feel unattractive and dispirited.

- Try to ensure that your child is not made to feel bad by having to take part in sports where she will always come last. Look for ways to exercise that are individual and where she can succeed. Encourage her to play sports that she likes and does well at.

- Don't nag about food or weight. Your child will resent you and withdraw, probably to a hidden stash of food.

- Be especially careful if you have a pre-teenage daughter. Our culture teaches young women to base their self-esteem almost solely on the shape and size of their bodies. If your daughter thinks you are criticizing her appearance, she may believe that you find her unacceptable too. She may deal with her crushed feelings by becoming anorexic in an effort to please you, or she may rebel and become even larger as an expression of anger and defiance.

- Instead of nagging, set a healthy example. Don't give one child a plate of 'diet' food while everyone else dives into pizza and chocolate cake. Make family meals healthy for everyone. Instead of collapsing in front of the TV after dinner, go for a walk or bike ride with the kids. At weekends take them hiking or introduce them to your favourite sport – but make sure you participate in it and don't just watch it on TV.

- In order to avoid rebellion and crushed feelings, when you talk to your children, focus on health, not appearance. Emphasize more activity, not less food. Diets create feelings of deprivation. For that reason they don't work for adults – and they won't work for kids either.

- Be realistic about your child's weight. Genes do make a difference. If a child is chubby but eats healthy foods in reasonable amounts, and if she is active and has self-control, she may be genetically predisposed to be heavier than average. Research suggests that this kind of extra weight is not as much of a health risk as the kind acquired via too many snack foods and too many hours on the internet. Just make sure they understand that personal worth depends on character, not on appearance.

- Find out if emotional stress or unhappiness is contributing to your child's weight gain. Children may substitute food for friends when they are lonely. They can also overeat when they are bored, angry, depressed, anxious, or otherwise stressed. If you suspect your child is eating in an attempt to numb painful feelings or escape stress, talk to your child and try to work out how to tackle the underlying cause of the problem, not just the symptom of eating. If you feel out of your depth, you may find it helpful to consult a qualified counsellor (see Resources page 251). Your doctor may also be able to refer your child to a counsellor.

- Food can take on emotional significance when used to comfort or reward children. It is, therefore, very important that you do not use food to comfort a child – listen to them patiently and give attention and hugs instead. Similarly, avoid using food as a reward as this can reinforce the idea of food as a source of comfort. Instead of having a fast-food meal to celebrate a good school report, for example, buy a gift, go to the cinema, or let them have a friend to stay overnight.

- A child may have turned to food and eating to somehow affect or camouflage feelings and emotions. In such cases, dysfunctional eating patterns become 'solutions' for real problems – but, of course, they create more problems, not fewer. It's extremely important that you identify problems that might be affecting your child, and teach him coping skills that do not involve foods (see page 192).

- When emotional issues are instrumental in your child becoming overweight, the emotional arena is obviously the first place to seek solutions and bring about change. It is a parent's responsibility to step in to encourage their child to recognize, define and resolve underlying emotional issues that may be driving their dysfunctional behaviours.

- It is a parent's responsibility to supply healthy meals regularly for children, and then to sit down to eat these meals together, listening to their child's thoughts and feelings at the same time as observing their eating behaviour. Children learn to like what they are accustomed to eating and what they see others eating. You may encounter some backlash at the beginning, but in the end, if mealtimes focus on positive conversation, there will be less of a battle about what is actually being served.

- Engage in activities, sports and healthy exercise with your child. Perhaps you might want to go for a bike ride together with your child, take tennis lessons together, or walk to the library, rather than drive. This will teach your child that you not only enjoy her company and want to spend time with her, but that you are involved in the process of changing lifestyle habits together. Everyone feels better when they have a partner in battle and your child will feel that she has all-important support. Furthermore, you are showing your child that you believe that exercise is part of a healthy lifestyle if you actively participate. There's no point in setting out a whole load of changes for your child that you do not show any interest in yourself.

- Although it sounds simplistic, what you need to remember is to focus on health, not appearance, and on more activity, not less food.

- Become alert to any stress your child might be experiencing at school or with peers. Remember that any form of extreme behaviour is unhealthy and may indicate anxiety. It is not uncommon for kids to attempt to soothe anxiety and solve problems through the use and abuse of food.

- Talk to your overweight child about whether he has ever experienced teasing in the schoolyard and, if so, discuss how he felt about it, and what he did or might do in response in the future. In Chapter 8 we'll look at ways to deal with bullying. This can be crucial in promoting self-esteem and teaching your child coping skills.

- To help your child, you need to understand what triggered his overeating and weight gain. First of all, you need to pinpoint when it started. Did it coincide with the death of someone he loved? The loss of a familiar babysitter? A separation or divorce in the family? The birth of a sibling? An illness or hospitalization? Bullying or stress at school? Any one of these events can emotionally disrupt a child's development, causing a change in eating habits. This change then initiates a vicious cycle: the more weight your child gains, the worse he feels about himself, and the worse he feels about himself, the more he turns to food for solace.

- How you talk about your child's body has a big impact on your child's self-image. Talk in terms of your child's health, activity level and other healthy lifestyle choices, rather than what she looks like. It's certainly important to acknowledge her concerns about feeling overweight, and the parts of her body that bother her, but it's easy to point out that everyone has bits of their bodies that they find unacceptable, and that everyone would like to be 'perfect'. No-one is perfect, of course, and teaching

A REALISTIC BODY IMAGE

Don't bother painting a picture of your child's body that is patently untrue. He'll see straight through your efforts and although he may appreciate them, he will never learn to trust what you say to him. There is no doubt that our society fosters the idea that we should all be a perfect size and weight, with long legs, slim waists, well-defined muscles and glowing skin and hair. The reality is that children – like adults – come in all shapes and sizes and 'perfection' is a fairly impossible goal, unless you resort to plastic surgery.

Children do need to learn that it is what is inside a person that matters, not just their appearance, and that some of the most popular and attractive people are not 'perfect' according to the current ideal. A good sense of humour, compassion, friendliness, happiness and honesty are all hugely attractive characteristics, and it is these that you want to foster in your child.

Children also need to feel good in their own skins – no matter what they look like. There is no point in overlooking an obvious weight problem that affects their appearance. Children are not blind, and they will feel ashamed if you do not show a willingness to discuss their concerns. Be honest with your child – agree that losing a little weight around her waist might make her skirt look better, but point out that if you work together on a more healthy lifestyle, she'll soon grow into her weight and look a lot slimmer. Forget about the idea of losing weight as a goal, as it will only create unhealthy habits (see page 130 The Object of Eating Well). Draw attention to the most attractive parts of her body, and help her to take pride in them. All

children that lesson is an important part of encouraging them to develop a healthy view of their bodies. Focus on her good points – hair, skin, a slimmer waist for example – if she hates how she looks, but lay the focus more on the good person she is, and the qualities that you admire about her personality and her approach to life.

- Be a good role model. Even if you struggle with how you feel about your own body, avoid talking about 'being fat' and 'needing to diet' in front of your child. Instead, talk about and make the same healthy lifestyle choices you'd like for your child.

children – and adults – have to accept their bodies at some point, and the happiest people are those who can see the good in themselves, without being overly concerned about perceived flaws. Once a child has reached puberty you can teach her to make the most of her best assets – show how you make your legs look longer by wearing a certain type of trousers, or minimize a slightly tubby waistline by wearing fitted t-shirts. Explain that a little tummy, curvy hips and breasts are part of becoming a woman, and that being womanly is much nicer than looking like a waif. Boys, too, need to know that they aren't born with a six-pack on their abdomens and that a little weight gain in puberty is very normal. Kids need to see that not all of us are designed perfectly, and that the best way to get on with things is to make the most of what we do have.

Some children have a completely distorted body image – slim young girls entering puberty, for example, may suddenly feel fat and actually believe they have a weight problem because they don't look exactly like their peers or their film-star heroines. It's very important that you nip this in the bud as early as possible, by explaining how bodies change as we grow older, and by pointing out that almost no-one in the 'real' world looks like the average teen role model. Teach a child to take pride in her body – again, focusing on the particularly attractive parts so that she is confident enough to overlook the less-than-perfect parts.

Finally, however, bear in mind that the most important thing that we can teach our children is that the people we are makes us more attractive than our physical appearance.

- Encourage social involvement in community and school activities, which build social skills and confidence.

Raising self-esteem and encouraging self-respect

Parents can have a direct impact on their children's self-esteem, so it is worth looking at how you interact with your children on a daily basis. A child with low self-esteem is not necessarily the product of poor parenting. There are many factors in this big, bad world that can affect the way your child views himself, but from the very first words you utter to your child, you can encourage or discourage a positive self-image.

When a child is born, he trusts his parents completely. Everything you say will be taken seriously. He will believe you. When parents are angry, upset, frustrated, busy or just exhausted, things come out that we don't intend. We label our children – you are stupid, frustrating, slow, an impossible eater, the worst sleeper – all kinds of things that just slip out. This is obviously the source of much parental guilt, and we often try to make it up with kisses and cuddles and even apologies later. But stop and consider this: your child believes everything you say. If you tell him he is stupid, even in a burst of anger, he will believe you. If you tell him he is selfish, he will think it's true. Every time we use negative words to define our children, they take them on board and file them away for future reference. No child will remember a particular incident, or be traumatized for life by being called stupid, but these occasions form faulty bricks in the foundation of his self-image. No matter how much you try to make up for it afterwards, if you have said something, your child believes it, even if it is at an unconscious level.

Consider the impact on a child with a weight problem. Anything negative that slips out will create an even lower self-opinion, and confirm his worst fears that he is not very worthy. Many parents of overweight kids also become frustrated when their children continue to put on weight despite their best efforts to curb the trend, and may snap or say things they don't mean, such as 'you'd be a lot thinner if you'd listen to what I said' or 'do you really need that food?' These little throwaway comments, even if they are not meant, can have a dramatic effect on the way your child perceives himself and the way he feels.

No parent can always be completely calm, or consistently show a level of self-control approaching sainthood, particularly with children about. What we need to do, however, is learn to think about how we say things in order to prevent labels from becoming self-fulfilling prophecies.

The importance of praise

Every adult knows how good it feels to be praised and in our society there is far too little of it. Everyone is too busy to stop and appreciate, to comment on the little things that make us feel good about ourselves. However, for any child, and particularly one with low self-esteem, praise can be invaluable.

Look back at your child's day. How often did you praise her? How did you make her feel good about herself? You might not have at all. If she was overexcited, grumpy or 'difficult', you probably blasted her. She may well have been disciplined, but she probably wasn't praised. Praise produces that warm feeling inside that makes your child think: I'm alright. She learns to feel good about herself, to appreciate and to see good in the world around her. She feels loved, valued and worthy of your attention. She sees that she can do good and that you will recognize it, and her, for her efforts. She learns to like herself and she develops confidence.

Fit praise into your day as often as you can – don't just concentrate on one area. If you only praise good marks, she may become obsessed with schoolwork as a way to please you. If you only praise her efforts on the hockey pitch, she may drive herself too hard to get your attention. If you never praise your child, she will continue to do whatever gets your attention, which probably means 'naughty' behaviour. And in the case of overweight children, this can be a rebellious attempt to eat more just to get the attention this undoubtedly brings.

From morning to night, notice and dwell on the good things about your child's behaviour – his actions, his personality and his views. That's not to say you should go overboard or be false; children see straight through false praise. Instead, recognize effort, achievement, good qualities and ideas your child has. Show interest and pride. Show an interest in him and his world. Be thrilled by his achievements, even if they don't live up to your expectations. If your child gets a report card full of Cs, but his teacher says he's really trying, make a fuss. If your child fails everything, but he gets a glowing personal report, focus on the fact that he is a nice, popular child. Praise everything good about your child and what he does. If he feels good about himself, if he believes you like him, flaws and all, he will develop self-esteem that will spill over into every part of his life. This is very important in an overweight child. They need to feel that they are successful in other areas in their lives, even if their bodies don't live up to their own expectations.

CASE HISTORY: ## Paul

During his first set of GCSE exams, Paul was under enormous pressure, both from his school and from his parents. He'd always been a perfectionist and was determined to prove that he was top of the class, and a candidate for a good university. But as the exams drew closer, he was not spending enough time revising. Instead, he spent hours on the computer and began to overeat for comfort. Even he couldn't understand why he wasn't making the effort he should. When the exam results came in, Paul had done very badly, which made him feel even worse about himself, and his overeating continued. Over a three-month period, he put on almost 13 kg (2 stone), and lost interest in anything other than the computer. His parents were at a loss to explain his change in behaviour.

On the advice of his doctor, Paul was referred to a counsellor, and depression was diagnosed. Over time, Paul grew to understand that his procrastination, not his ability, was the reason for his poor results. He also realized that the reason for his procrastination lay in his fear of failure, of not making the mark, even though he was perfectly capable of getting the good grades he had always achieved. He began to see that his eating habits had developed as a form of comfort, and that he felt happier and better when he ate. Through perseverance and several months of counselling, he took his own diet in hand, and with the support of his teachers, decided to focus on his A levels. He began a regular revision programme, with plenty of time for exercise and fun with his friends, and began to see that he had been his own worst enemy by putting too much pressure on himself.

Paul is due to sit his exams shortly and already feels much more confident and back to his old self. His coursework grades have been consistently good, and regular exercise with friends has given him another focus to his life. He's back to his fighting weight, too, as he has been far too active to need food to fill a hole in his life.

Most importantly, however, praise your child for just being himself. Praise his appearance (you are such a good-looking boy, your hair looks nice today, you've got such a great smile, you look good in those jeans, what gorgeous eyes…). Although an emphasis on appearance is a definite 'no-no' when it comes to raising kids with a healthy self-image and lots of confidence, even overweight children need to know that they are attractive and have features that are perfectly lovely.

As I've said before, children will define their bodies by how others perceive them. If you make them feel that they are attractive, you will improve their confidence and their self-image. Fat children, skinny children, adolescents with acne – everyone needs to feel that they are loveable and nice to look at. You won't create a big-headed child by praising their appearance, you'll simply ensure that your child feels comfortable in his own skin.

Physical affection

Nurturing touch plays a strong role in infant and child development and research suggests that it continues to be important as a way of communicating love and caring between parents and their older children. Most parents continue to share some level of physical closeness with their daughters during the teenage years, but this can change dramatically for sons. Most parents (mothers in particular) of boys find that this nurturing physical contact with a son grows more awkward and less frequent by around the age eight or nine, but the shift is perhaps most dramatic when he moves into adolescence. Many children naturally withdraw, particularly in front of their friends, and this is something we have to expect and respect. However, it doesn't mean that we should give it up altogether. Like many other aspects of parenting, physical closeness remains important throughout a child's life. As they get older, parents are among the few people who can give a child the emotional comfort of physical warmth in a non-sexual context, and children need to experience physical tenderness if they are to be able to be physical themselves as adults.

A child who is not touched will feel ignored, ashamed, unworthy of attention and unhappy. There are many studies that reflect the power of touch (babies, for example, thrive better when there is physical contact), and we need to remember that touch is important throughout childhood and into adolescence and beyond. Touch has a language of its own. It can offer reassurance and love that goes beyond words. A pat on the shoulder, a warm embrace, a gentle massage, tousling hair or stroking a much-loved little

SELF-RESPECT

The most important quality with which you can imbue your child is self-respect. It differs from self-esteem in several key ways. The first is that respect means a conscious understanding of strong points and limitations. It means accepting themselves as they are, not as some perfect child with expectations to live up to and an unreal sense of their own capabilities and weaknesses. While esteem is awarded, respect must be earned through responsibility, cooperation and achievement. If we avoid the use of self-respect and substitute self-esteem, we have a convenient way of avoiding the effort required to succeed. For example, giving everyone a trophy simply because they participated in a race would increase everyone's self-esteem, but not their self-respect.

When a child learns to respect himself, he also learns the ability to respect others – and other things, such as property, motivation, emotions, responsibility and authority. The reason is that he has earned his self-image and he can respect that. The process that led him there will be etched in his mind, and he will be able to draw upon that in different situations throughout his life, when dealing with others and when acting in society as a whole. A child with respect for himself has a much clearer view of his own strengths and weaknesses and can accept them. This is incredibly important in the context of an overweight child. Many children with weight problems lack the self-respect necessary to respect their bodies. No-one else seems to show them any respect, so they don't have any themselves. They also have a tendency to focus on their weaknesses rather than seeing them as an acceptable part of the person they are – an imperfection, perhaps, in some people's eyes, but part of what makes them them and unique. A child with self-respect can accept weaknesses and focus on strengths – and, most importantly, play on those strengths and use them to achieve what they want from their lives.

You can't 'give' your child self-respect, but you can ensure that he earns it by offering him opportunities to take responsibility; by giving him unqualified attention and unconditional love (hence enhancing his belief in himself as a unique individual, worthy of such attention); by providing realistic goals and praising their attainment; by rewarding genuine effort and achievement rather than blindly praising things that show no enterprise, initiative or effort; by encouraging him to feel good about himself and his body; by praising the things that make him special; and by teaching respect for others, so that he can find the same qualities that he respects within himself.

face can communicate acceptance and affection that tell your child how you feel about him. Be careful, however, not to demand affection when *you* need it. Watch for signs that your child needs a little reassurance – and make it natural. An attention-seeking child may need a little of just that – quality attention. Sit down together with a book and put your arm around your child. If he's watching television, stroke his feet. If he's struggling with homework, give him a hug. Get down there and be physical. There is safety in physical affection, and all children will benefit.

This brings us to the question of bodies. Children need to feel good about their bodies and themselves, and physical affection can provide reassurance that they are attractive and loveable. No-one touches things that they find distasteful and if you fail to touch your child, he will get the message that he is something with which you would rather not be in contact – even if this is on a subconscious level. Touch raises self-esteem and makes children feel good about their bodies.

Quiz

How is your child's emotional health?
Answer the following questions honestly:
1. Can your child tell you how he is genuinely feeling? (This doesn't mean coming out with a pat 'I'm sad', or 'I'm happy' in response to your questions. It means that your child can express his feelings – at bedtime, in a quiet moment, or in the throes of an argument – without being pushed to do so.)
2. Does your child exhibit signs of stress (see page 243)?
3. Does your child seem listless or withdrawn on a regular basis?
4. Does your child laugh less than he used to?
5. Does your child smile or show delight easily?
6. Does your child become frustrated easily, and want to give up?
7. Does your child push himself too hard – to be the best, the top of the class, the best player on the pitch, or the winner of the prize?
8. Is your child reluctant to take on new challenges or activities that he would normally enjoy?

9. Does your child become extremely upset if criticized or corrected?
10. Does your child put himself down regularly?
11. Is your child overly critical of others?
12. Does your child try too hard to please people (teachers, friends, family members)?
13. Is your child clingy?
14. Does your child suffer from inexplicable fears, or is he afraid to face new situations?
15. Does your child need continual approval?
16. Does your child boast?
17. Is your child aggressive or attention seeking?
18. Is your child impatient and unappreciative?
19. Does your child suffer from a series of low-grade infections, abdominal pains or headaches that cannot be explained, but appear regularly?

Interpreting the result

If you answered yes to the first question and no to all the others, you have a supremely balanced child and you are unlikely to need to read this chapter. Chances are, however, that you will have a combination of yes and no answers. This isn't a test, but it provides a basis for understanding the signs of emotional imbalance, which can impact on your child's life in many ways. An overweight child will undoubtedly have some emotional issues affecting or causing their weight problem, and working out periods when your child is particularly prone can help to pinpoint their cause. Emotional imbalance in children does not automatically indicate poor parenting; today's children are under stress in a variety of ways. There is no need to be ashamed or embarrassed if your child is struggling emotionally. Simply use it as a cue to make changes that will make her feel better about herself, and more able to cope with the world around her.

What you need to do is try to ensure that your child is emotionally balanced, so that she feels good about herself, feels confident in new situations, doesn't feel a need to be the best or to get the most, or look perfect, is patient and, above all, likes herself. No child will ever be or look perfect, and there will always be times when she experiences dips in confidence, has feelings of low self-worth, loses her temper and lashes out, and even becomes depressed. Like physical health, emotional health can slip and soar. In the same way that you can take steps to boost your child's physical health through a healthy diet and lifestyle, you can boost your child's emotional health, to help her get through the multitude of new situations that will face her throughout her life.

Emotional support

According to Karen DeBord, PhD, a child development specialist, parents have an important role to play in helping children to cope with stress, difficult periods in their lives and emotional difficulties. She says, 'Just as children's reactions are each different, so are their coping strategies. Children can cope through tears or tantrums or by retreating from unpleasant situations. They could be masterful at considering options, finding compromising solutions, or finding substitute comfort. Usually a child's thinking is not developed fully enough to think of options or think about the results of possible actions. Children who live in supportive environments and develop a range of coping strategies become more resilient. Resiliency is the ability to bounce back from stress and crisis. For many children, a supportive environment is not present and many children do not learn a set of positive coping strategies.'

She believes that families can help their children by:
- Developing trust, particularly during the first year of life
- Being supportive
- Showing caring and warmth
- Having high, clear expectations without being overly rigid
- Providing ways for children to contribute to the family in meaningful ways
- Building on family strengths.

Acceptance

What children need most from their parents is unconditional love and acceptance, which gives them the courage and strength to explore, take risks, challenge, attempt and achieve the things they want in life. A child who is accepted can be more realistic about her shortcomings and her strengths and develop self-respect (see page 186). An overweight child who is accepted for who she is will not develop an unhealthy obsession with her weight, and will be able to deal clearly and confidently with the problem.

Do you offer emotional support to your child? If so, in what way? Do you accept the good with the bad, the failures with the successes? If your approach to parenting focuses too heavily on judging your child, on discipline, behaviour, achievement, performance, appearance and fulfilling expectations, your child will not have the support she needs to deal with stressful situations, and she will not have the communication channel she needs to express concerns, learn from failure, and, ultimately, know that there is someone, somewhere, who will love her no matter what she does or what she looks like.

If a child lives with encouragement and appreciation, she becomes confident. If her main relationships are with people who are patient and undemanding, she will develop the security to try new things without a fear of failure. She will not be afraid of failing to live up to expectations, and she will be encouraged to celebrate successfully reaching personal goals – all of which makes her stronger and more resilient to peer pressure, life's ups and downs and all the knocks along the way. If a child feels good about herself, and is supported in that belief, she will meet challenges with vigour and enthusiasm. Most importantly, however, she will be happy. And a happy child is in a much stronger position to deal with weight problems if and when they crop up. She'll have self-belief, coping skills, the emotional energy to tackle a problem and the motivation to look and feel her best.

Time and interaction

We've already established that children have far too little meaningful time with their parents, even in families who make a concerted effort to spend time together. Struggles over homework, rushing to activities, grabbing a quick dinner and scrabbling to prepare for the next day do not produce a climate conducive to interaction and sharing. Children need to be encouraged to talk, and adults need to find or make the time in which to do just that. Asking the same questions of your child at the end of every day, in your half an hour of allotted 'quality time', will not produce genuine and positive communication. Children will tune out, or reluctantly recite the events that took place that day.

Converse with your child in much the same way as you would a friend, bringing up interesting situations or elements of your own day, or asking their opinion about a piece of news or even a new colour for the sitting-room wall. Ask them interesting, focused questions that are relevant to their state of mind, their mood and their activities. This doesn't mean treating them like adults, it simply means giving them the respect that you give to adults. 'What did you have for lunch?' is never going to inspire stimulating conversation, nor is an unhealthy focus on the day's test results. Ask questions that you know will interest him, and take an interest in his interests! Find out the latest team line-up for a match he wants to watch, bone up on the group he's into, find out some good gossip about something that interests him and you'll get the ball rolling. Once the channels of communication are open, you'll establish the type of relationship where chatting, revealing and confiding are commonplace – and you'll find that a certain level of trust is also established.

Communication is one of the most important elements of emotional health, yet the majority of children simply do not confide in their parents, either because they fear recrimination or they never have a genuine opportunity to do so.

Time is the crucial element here and you simply have to be prepared to make it. If children grow up never forming strong bonds with close family and friends, never sharing problems or working on solutions and coping strategies, they are unlikely to do so in adulthood, which is a very unhealthy situation indeed.

As you will by now be aware, one of the keys to assessing a child's weight problem is to work out what emotional factors may have triggered it, or be exacerbating it. If you don't talk to your child and rarely spend time with her, you'll be unlikely to find out that cause. It's also unlikely that you'll have the kind of relationship necessary to foster changes. Your child needs to be able to talk to you, to listen when you explain solutions to problems; they need to receive understanding and be able to feel that they can come to you with any problems that crop up. Many children with weight problems feel isolated, and drawing such a child closer into the family unit can make a big difference. Sneaky habits, comfort eating and unhealthy associations with food are much less likely to take place if the family unit is strong and you are there for your child when she needs you. Instead of using food in the place of love and reassurance, she'll have the real thing.

Coping skills

A large part of a parent's job is to help their children develop coping skills – tactics that will enable them to get through situations that present a challenge or a problem. You'll need to use your antennae for this one because it may not always be evident when there is a problem. When you have established good communication, you will hopefully find yourself the recipient of news both good and bad, and you can gauge where problems might lie.

Children simply do not have the tools, the insight, the experience or the confidence to face every problem on their own. Part of life is learning how to deal with different people and situations, and parents need to be involved along the way, to ensure that little things aren't becoming insurmountable issues. Tell your child about a similar experience that happened to you when you were a child. Ensure that your child feels that his situation and his response are absolutely normal. Never demand a brave face, or suggest that he deal with it on his own. The best way for children to learn to cope is by offering a variety of different suggestions from which they can choose the most appropriate. They'll then feel in control, plus they'll be much more likely to ask your advice in future, as well as feeling much more confident about their coping skills in general.

And in the context of a weight problem, this is critical. Many overweight children feel out of control and really do not know how to deal with the emotions they are experiencing, or their cravings for foods, or the sneaking suspicion that their relationship with food is not normal. They might know they have a problem but that doesn't mean they have any idea how to go about changing things. However, many parents shove the issues under the carpet rather than acknowledging a child's concerns and offering a real solution

CASE HISTORY: Bella

Bella began to put on weight when she was about to enter primary school, at a time when her parents were getting divorced. The divorce led to a house move and a new partner for her dad. Her parents indulged her a little and allowed her to indulge herself in treats that were not normally allowed. The result was a significant weight gain, which affected her self-esteem and made her draw into herself. Her mother was struggling to get over the break-up of her marriage, while her dad was involved with his new partner, and so the problem was constantly overlooked. Bella didn't feel that she had anyone to turn to – she didn't want to add to her mother's problems and her dad just didn't seem to be there for her anymore. Hers was a classic case of a child experiencing neglect, which contributed to her problem.

When a school nurse drew attention to Bella's weight her parents were forced to take note, and Bella was angry and upset enough to spill the beans. When it became clear that her problem had an emotional basis, her parents overcame their hostility towards one another and jointly developed a programme to get her back on track. Bella's mum stopped focusing on her own problems and spent more time with Bella, and her dad agreed to spend a day a week with her – on her own, and without his new partner around, as well as undertaking regular visits – to give her the quality time she needed. They encouraged her to open up and helped her deal with her new situation by being loving and patient. As a result, Bella soon lost the need to turn to food for comfort and over the coming year, her weight balanced out.

to problems. Again, this serves to make a child feel alone and frightened. And children in this position do not have the resource necessary to cope. So little problems become big ones, and once again they turn to food for comfort and reassurance.

What we are aiming for is resilience. Drs Robert Brooks and Sam Goldstein founded the Raising Resilient Children Project to help adults to raise, support and develop emotionally hardy children. They say, 'Resilience embraces the ability of a child to deal more effectively with stress and pressure, to cope with everyday challenges, to bounce back from disappointments, adversity and trauma, to develop clear and realistic goals to solve problems, to relate comfortably to others and to treat oneself and others with respect. Numerous scientific studies of children facing adversity in their lives have supported the importance of resilience as a powerful insulating force. Resilience explains why some children overcome overwhelming obstacles, sometimes clawing and scraping their way to successful adulthood while others become victims of their early experiences and environments.'

They also stress the importance of empathy in communication with our children. They believe that empathy is a starting point to help children locate areas of competence and success in their lives, to develop problem-solving skills, responsibility, compassion and a social conscience. In their words, 'Empathy permits us to communicate the message to our children that we hear, feel, and understand their opinions; it helps us to find ways to validate what our children are saying and attempting to accomplish. This does not imply that we agree with everything our children think, believe or do but rather that we acknowledge what they are saying.'

If your child's concerns are heard, and he feels that he has your support and guidance, he will be much more likely to confide in you, which gives you the opportunity to develop strategies to deal with problems as they arise. Children who learn at a young age to deal with problems, or to become more resilient, are those who have developed coping skills along the way. Rather than retiring to their rooms, giving up the things that will make and keep them healthy, such as exercise, a good night's sleep and a healthy diet, and turning to food for comfort, children can rely on themselves (often with the support of their

SELF-ESTEEM

Self-esteem can be defined as the combination of feelings of capability with feelings of being loved. A child who is happy with her achievements but does not feel loved may eventually experience low self-esteem. Likewise, a child who feels loved but is hesitant about her own abilities can also end up feeling negatively about herself. Healthy self-esteem results when the right balance is attained.

families) to get through problem periods – many of which are a natural part of growing up – and to find solutions that work for them.

Your family dynamic

The essential ingredient in any happy family is love: unconditional love. Erich Fromm, the famous psychologist and philosopher, once wrote that 'unconditional love corresponds to one of the deepest longings, not only of the child, but of every human being.' In today's chaotic world, where time is at a premium, this foundation-stone of unconditional love can ensure a happy family relationship, one that all family members benefit from and grow within.

Quiz

How healthy is your family relationship?

1 Does everyone in the family have an equal voice and recognition?
2 Do you feel that your family members respect one another and you?
3 Do all family members take pride in the others' achievements?
4 Do you have a family system for recognizing achievement?
5 Do you eat together as a family at least three times a week?
6 Do you share family activities at least three times a week?
7 Does every family member have time to be alone?
8 Does every family member have separate interests, activities and hobbies, with time allowed to undertake them?
9 Does your family watch less than five hours of television a week?
10 Does everyone in the family have responsibilities?
11 Is your family environment calm and loving?
12 Do all family members cope well with stress?
13 Does your family laugh a lot?
14 Does your child feel comfortable bringing friends home to play or visit?
15 Do leisure activities play an important role in family life?
16 Does your family have extended family members in close, regular contact?
17 Is everyone in good physical health?

Interpreting the result

If you can answer yes to all of these questions, the family environment you are providing for your child sounds perfect. The object of this exercise is, however, to find areas of weakness. For questions to which you have answered 'no', consider why. All of these elements are part of a happy family life, and will affect the way your child grows, learns, views the world and, ultimately, copes with problems both now and in the future. By understanding weaknesses in the family dynamic, you can take steps to address them – all of which will benefit your child. An overweight child with a healthy family unit is much less likely to become obese, or to resort to comfort eating or binge eating/dieting when facing problems. She'll have a strong foundation, and someone to turn to when the going gets tough.

Food and mood

No discussion of emotional health would be complete without considering the effect that food has on mood. Many of your child's feelings may, in fact, be linked to what he eats, which is one reason why changing your family diet is not just important in the battle to control weight, but essential to health in the long run – on both a physical and emotional level.

It's easy to see the impact poor nutrition has on kids. Consider your child's state of mind after a party where there are loads of sugary, refined foods. They are often tearful, fussy, tired and fractious. Their physical health in this case has impacted upon their emotional well-being. Think of times when they haven't had enough sleep – their behaviour and their moods change. That's because the physical and mental functions are interlinked.

Your child's diet may make him feel tired, headachy and irritable. Too much caffeine may mean that his sleep is not as restful as it should be, that he can't settle down at a reasonable time, or that he wakens frequently. Too many sweets, junk foods and carbohydrates may cause surges in blood sugar that lead to hyperactivity, and then a subsequent drop that causes feelings of depression and low mood, as well as an overwhelming exhaustion. Lack of concentration is also a common feature of a poor diet, and your child's grades may be affected, which compounds feelings of inadequacy or low self-worth.

SIGNS OF AN EMOTIONALLY BALANCED CHILD

- A strong relationship with at least one parent or close adult
- Well-developed social skills
- Well-developed problem-solving skills
- An ability to act independently
- A sense of purpose and of the future
- At least one coping strategy
- A sense of positive self-esteem and personal responsibility
- Ability to focus attention
- Special interests and hobbies.

Does your child have these? Stress, low self-esteem, problems at school, worries about weight and a poor body image affect all of these characteristics, but all of this can be improved and attained with the love and support of a healthy family unit, whether there is one parent, two working parents, or the traditional one-income family.

Studies also show that carbohydrate cravers experience amazing lows and obese carbohydrate cravers often score high on tests for depression. When participants in one study were asked why they eat so much food, knowing it would exacerbate their obesity, they responded that it is rarely connected to hunger or taste – these foods helped them feel calm and reduced anxiety. When carbohydrate cravers and non-cravers were fed a carbohydrate-rich meal, the cravers' mood was improved for up to three hours after eating and they were less depressed after eating, while the non-cravers reported fatigue and sleepiness. For more information on this problem, see page 80.

A poor diet can also lead to nutritional deficiencies that affect brain chemistry and the efficiency of every body system. This can't fail to impact on behaviour and mood – when one part of our body is out of kilter, the other parts follow suit.

So even before you take steps to change your family dynamic, and to boost your child's self-esteem and self-image, ensure that you get his diet right. Fresh, whole foods, with few additives, sugar, caffeine, refined and processed ingredients, will kick-start the whole process by helping to ensure that your child's emotional health is not being negatively affected by what she eats.

It's very clear that there are many aspects of our children's lifestyle that will affect their emotional health and the way they feel about themselves. While this chapter may represent a long list of changes that you feel you must make to your family unit, and the way you interact with your child, the effort you make will be more than worthwhile. For one thing, all family members will benefit from a happier family dynamic and a more hands-on approach to parenting. Secondly, even if your child's weight problem is short-lived she will have a much stronger emotional foundation to deal with problems in the future, and to cope with difficulties that may cause her to overeat.

In conclusion

No parent can argue that spending more time together and working on strengthening relationships between family members is a wasted effort. Our job is to send our children into the world brimming with confidence and self-belief, feeling good about their bodies and their minds, recognizing their strengths and their weaknesses, and able to express their emotions. Happy, healthy children are those that are emotionally balanced, and weight problems are far less likely to be an issue for a child who feels good and in control. If you can get to the root of an emotional problem in your child, deal with any issues she has with food and comfort, give her love and a secure family unit to fall back upon (and it doesn't matter how big that family is; a family of two is still a unit), and combine this with a good strong family policy on healthy eating, leisure and exercise, you'll have covered all the key risk factors for overweight and obesity, and be well on your way to solving the problem.

Chapter Seven

A Little Extra Help

Even the best-laid plan can go awry from time to time, and there is certainly no shame in admitting that you need some help. It can be very difficult to convince children, particularly pre-teenagers and teenagers, of the necessity of broad-scale changes. Faddy eaters and junk-food addicts, games console junkies and exercise phobics may also challenge your patience when you lay down new rules and ways of operating as a family. It's also worth remembering that many overweight children will have suffered a battering to their self-esteem and confidence, and may use your new regime as an excuse for rebellion or self-pity. It's not easy changing a lifestyle, even if you know that it is the right thing to do.

What's more, some children may be seriously overweight or obese, and suffer withdrawal symptoms from the foods they can no longer eat, and a serious crisis of confidence when faced with the prospect of undertaking a more active lifestyle. Long-term habits can be hard to shift, and kids are not always open to change.

It is important to remember that they will, eventually, come round and if you undertake the same changes yourself, and become a good role model for your children, they will learn through example and the changes will become habit as a matter of course. But it can take time and you may need some support along the way. Parents of overweight kids are often the target of abuse, as well, and you may have had to cope with feelings of guilt and shame, inspired by the unkind comments of people who simply don't understand the reasons why children today are overweight. While you should, by now, be reassured that you are not solely to blame for your child's problem, it can be exhausting and demoralizing to be faced with criticism from ignorant people.

You may also have to deal with people who sabotage your efforts – dinner or cafeteria workers at school, well-meaning grandparents, your children's peers and even your children's own siblings. All of these things can undermine your patience and your determination to succeed.

This chapter examines how to cope with the problems that you might face when undertaking a new regime. We'll look at ways to deal with some of the particular problems that might be causing or accompanying your child's weight problem – issues such as blood sugar problems, food allergies, nutritional deficiencies, carbohydrate cravings and even depression. All of these can undermine your efforts if they are not treated alongside dietary and lifestyle changes.

Many parents will expect a fairly dramatic response to a big family change, and may be disappointed to discover that there is no quick-fix solution – that it will take time, energy, effort, patience and determination to make the necessary changes, and even longer for your child to respond in terms of balancing his weight and growing into the extra weight that he has acquired.

A few children simply don't respond well at all, and you may need to seek the help of professionals in order to put together a solution that will work for your individual child. The vast majority of children will, however, see some dramatic changes to their overall health and well-being, so don't be tempted to give up. A little fine-tuning here and there, along the way, may be necessary to make it work for your child, but overall, you will see changes, even if they take some time to become clear.

Inspiring your child

Your overweight child may not want to admit that she has a problem, or she may feel concerned about making changes that make her feel different to her peers, or singled out because there is something wrong with her. One of the premises of this book is that you do not need to draw attention to a weight problem in order to make these changes. In fact, if you make a child feel that they have a problem, you may undermine their self-esteem further and fail to gain their support. You may face rebellion, tantrums or even tears, which will make it difficult to encourage your child to try something new. So the new programme is all about change – for health, a better family dynamic and a happier, healthier lifestyle that will benefit all family members. And to make the changes necessary to deal with weight problems, every family member does need to be involved. You aren't putting your child on a diet. You aren't changing his lifestyle. You are adapting the way your family lives, and that is the message that must be passed on for you to experience success.

Some children will be only too aware that they are overweight, and they may already have enlisted your support to help them lose weight – or change their shape. In this case, there is no point in dismissing their concerns. But you need to put the focus on the whole family rather than your overweight child. Make it clear that you understand his worries, but that you have realized that it is your family lifestyle and eating habits that are to blame rather than anything he has done. If you shift the blame, you free your child from the idea that he is alone in dealing with a problem, and even that he has a problem. It's a family issue and you'll deal with it together.

If your child does need a little help from a professional, or has an underlying problem, such as carbohydrate cravings or depression, you can gently suggest that you go to the doctor together to find out if there is anyone who can help him to feel better. For this reason, the issues that we discussed in the last chapter are extremely important – you need to open up the channels of communication so that your child can feel comfortable confiding in you and expressing his concerns. You must be patient, understanding and sympathetic. You must also expect some resistance – no child wants to be singled out and treated as if he is ill in some way. Broaching the subject of extra help means encouraging your child to come to the conclusion himself that a few new ideas or a little intervention might make things easier. Discuss the symptoms of various underlying problems, such as depression or blood sugar disorders, and ask him if they seem to be relevant to the way he is feeling. Make it clear that you want your child to be happy, and that you need a little help getting him there. Everything you say must be positive and geared towards making your child feel that you care enough to want the best for him.

In order to inspire your children and the rest of the family to make changes, you have to be prepared to explain why they are necessary. Throughout the book I've looked at all the problems associated with an unhealthy lifestyle and diet – including those that have nothing to do with weight. Look them up and use them. You are changing your diet because an unhealthy diet leads to heart disease, diabetes, tooth decay and some forms of cancer, and you want the best for your family. You need exercise to relieve stress, to sleep better, and to have better concentration and balanced moods. You don't like the type of advertising that litters most TV programmes, and you also know that too much TV can be unhealthy. You don't have to mention weight to get your message across.

Get excited! Explain that you've been doing some reading and you really feel that it's time for your family as a whole to shape up. You think you need more time together (and what child is going to object to more parental attention?) and less junk food. You want to get the whole family involved in some new hobbies – and some fun activities together. Be positive! Make it sound like a promising and rewarding prospect. Show that you understand that some changes might be hard to make at the beginning, but that they will make every family member feel better, look better, function better and experience a greater sense of well-being.

Enlisting support

There are two elements to the notion of enlisting support – support for your new programme, and support for you. You and your family will bear the responsibility of supporting your overweight child through the changes, and it's very important that you have both back-up and emotional assistance and encouragement as you do so.

Talk to a good friend about what you are trying to do, and try to choose a friend who understands the importance of a healthy diet. You need someone who will support you and not undermine your efforts because they feel guilty that they aren't doing the same with their own families. Make sure your partner is involved and understands the reasons for the change. You may find that he or she is reluctant to change eating habits or leisure activities to any great extent, but if you point out the dangers that your overweight child could

GET ANGRY, NOT ANXIOUS

The unbelievable flood of tempting goodies aimed at children, combined with the sophisticated marketing techniques used to sell them, means that such products are a powerful influence on the way our children eat. Their impact is hardly surprising when you consider the teams of food technologists, designers, psychologists and advertising executives employed by companies to create and market these products, the very products that are contributing to overweight in children. Bear this in mind and don't feel like a failure if your child spurns the healthy food you offer. Remember that the food designed to appeal to children has been created with kids in mind, and aimed at their perceived needs. In reality, few children can resist products endorsed by their favourite pop or sports stars – it encourages kids to feel that they are buying into pop culture. Cartoon characters, free gifts and competitions are also designed to draw children to products and keep them hooked. What's more, by using artificial colours and flavourings in foods created for children, manufacturers make poor-quality food look much more attractive than the healthier options.

It's a difficult task to encourage children to resist something that has been so carefully designed to attract them. Even armed with an understanding of nutrition and the problems that unhealthy foods can cause, the majority of children do not see these products as being unhealthy or unacceptable, because they are the norm in their peer group, they are endorsed by their idols and mentors, and they quite simply look much more tantalizing than anything that the average parent can produce at home. In addition, manufacturers have now cottoned on to the idea that kids are being pressured and educated to eat well, so they market unhealthy products as being healthier than they actually are. A few added vitamins or minerals, some natural fruit juice, or a lower sugar content encourage kids to believe that they are making an acceptable choice when, in reality, such ploys often simply disguise junk food. So what can you do? Get together with other parents to persuade the food industry to improve its products, and to put pressure on politicians to raise food standards. Groups like Parents Jury and The Food Commission in the UK evolved to do just this. So why not get involved? You too can add your voice to the growing number of parents who want to see the food industry clean up its act. (See Resources page 250 for details of these organizations.)

face, you should be able to get them on board. After a period of living well, every family member will feel the benefits, and it won't be long before changes become habit.

Getting support also means involving grandparents, carers, childminders, au pairs and anyone else who may look after your child. There is no point in making broad-scale adjustments to the way you live your life if some of the people, some of the time, allow old habits to rear their heads. Some carers might be reluctant to take on changes that create more work – particularly if they look after a lot of children. And the last thing you want to do is to draw attention to your child and single him out in front of others. If your carer is unwilling to change the foods she provides for the children she looks after, don't be tempted to send in 'special' food for your child, which will just make him stand out and feel that he has a problem, or that he is different. Instead, suggest that single helpings, smaller quantities and as few treats as possible be offered to your child. But take the time to explain why you are adopting new policies – and talk to the parents of other children, as well; they may be keen for their children to be involved, too. You may also have to outline the importance of some exercise and less TV for your child when you are not looking after him. A good carer will not rely on TV or computer games to occupy children, and most will plan at least some active pursuits in the course of a day. If this is not the case, it might be time to change carers.

Many grandparents like to spoil their grandchildren by giving them their favourite foods and extra treats, often against their parents' wishes – and as 'a little secret' between them and the children. You absolutely must make clear to all members of your family that they are not helping your child or you by doing this. Be firm, and explain to them the reality of overweight and the health problems that it could cause your child. Ask for their support and get them on your side. Some grandparents will not believe that a little 'puppy fat' on a beloved grandchild could really be a problem, and you may have to educate them. Take the time to do so. It's worth the effort. They may well feel flattered, too, that you need their help.

You can also write to – or visit, if necessary – school nurses, PE teachers, youth workers (even the head dinner lady if it'll help) in order to advise them of your plan to change things in order to balance your child's weight. Most people today are aware of the crises with overweight children, and will respect and appreciate your efforts. You may need to suggest that healthier options, such as lean meats or salad bars, be made available in the school canteen, or that chips are not served every day. You may not get anywhere, but it's worth a try. If you can find other likeminded parents, you may be able to gather enough support for changes to be made.

If your child takes a packed lunch, ask that there be a 'no swapping' policy, to prevent your child from eating the remains of another child's lunch. And, as I've said before, suggest that lunchboxes are not emptied before they are returned home, so that you can check what your child has eaten. If he's regularly leaving the fruit and veggies untouched, you'll need to put some rules into place.

Some schools are open to the idea of changing their snack and lunchbox policies, particularly in light of the growing trend towards obesity. Many schools now suggest that crisps and chocolate or sweets are not appropriate snacks, and even offer 'healthy' lunchbox ideas for parents. See if you can initiate such a policy in your child's school.

Older siblings may work out that the reason for the changes in your household are due to one or more family members being overweight, and may be resentful rather than supportive. It's very important that you ensure that no teasing takes place or any subversive comments are made. Make it clear that you are making changes for the benefit of the whole family. And that as a family, you will work together to make them happen. Explain your reasons, without pointing the finger at one child.

Talk to your doctor and, if necessary, ask to be referred to a dietitian, who can point you in the right direction if you're finding things difficult. If your request proves fruitless you can contact one privately (see Resources page 254). The guidance in this book will work for the vast majority of families, but if you have questions or concerns you might want to talk things over with an expert. This may also be necessary if your child is seriously obese and requires some professional help. It's also a good idea to talk through your concerns with your doctor if you believe your child's weight problems are linked to a serious emotional disorder, or if you suspect that there are underlying health problems. You may be referred to a counsellor or a specialist, such as an endocrinologist, for extra help. If you are finding things very difficult, your doctor may also be able to arrange for some support for you, such as nurse or counsellor, who can see you through any difficult periods.

Finding the patience and determination

Over the first few weeks and even months, your patience may be stretched to the limit, especially if your child suffers from difficult moods when his favourite foods are withdrawn or limited from the family dining table. You may find that your child refuses to help himself, and breaks the rules or eats sneakily at any opportunity. At times it may seem that all of your efforts are likely to be in vain. However, it's important to persevere. Slowly but surely, children do come round to different diets and ways of doing things, even if they resist at first. Their old eating habits will eventually become a distant memory. You may have to get tough from time to time, and insist that leisure activities do not include too much TV, that junk food does not appear in the house, and that physical activity does take place. Set up a reward system for effort and achievement. Continually encourage your child, even when you think your patience is about to snap. It can seem very unfair that you are doing your best to help a child who is resisting your efforts, but remember that you are dealing with a child, and you are ultimately in charge. Be firm but patient.

You will come across setbacks (see Chapter 8), but work through these sensitively and try to ascertain the root cause rather than just assuming your child is being rebellious. Overweight and obesity are, in some senses of the words, eating disorders and even lifestyle disorders, and the best way to deal with them is to be persistent but understanding. Climb straight back on the horse, and believe in what you are doing.

If you need motivation, re-read the introduction to this book, which outlines the very real dangers of overweight and obesity. Pick up a newspaper and see what's happening to children all around us, all over the world, as a result of these conditions. You want what is best for your child and, as a parent, it's your job to provide it. Bear that in mind, and stick to your principles.

Easing in a new regime

Some children will be literally addicted to a poor diet, and suffer the equivalent of withdrawal symptoms when you change what they are eating. This is often the case with children whose diet is very limited. Some signs of withdrawal include moodiness, edginess, trouble sleeping, tearfulness and, in extreme circumstances, shaking. Kids who have been drinking vast quantities of fizzy drinks, for example, may have become slightly dependent on a caffeine rush, and feel very out of sorts when it is cut from their diet.

If your child is experiencing these kinds of symptoms, you may need to ease them into a healthier way of eating. Cut down on the fizzy drinks a little each day, and do the same with favourite foods that they overeat. Over a period of two weeks or so, symptoms should abate – even if they do go 'cold turkey'. Remember why they are feeling this way, explain to them that what they are experiencing is normal, and a pretty good sign that changes were necessary – no-one wants to be an addict! Again, be patient and help your child to get through difficult periods. Offer your support and understanding, but persevere.

Dealing with blame and guilt

Too often parents are given the blame for having an overweight child, when there are many, many factors behind the problem. Most of us do what we think is best for our children as they grow up, and are aghast to find that we may have been misguided, or we took our eye off the ball for longer than we should have done. That doesn't make us bad parents, in any sense of the word. You may have overfed your child out of love, and because it made him feel good when he was given treats and extra goodies. You may have fallen into the trap of using food for comfort – something almost every parent does from time to time. You may have allowed sedentary habits to develop because you've been busy and it was often impossible to nudge your child into action. You may have resisted a battle to keep a modicum of peace in the family. Whatever the reasons may be, you did not knowingly, or willingly, encourage your child to become fat.

So taking the blame for something you did not intend can be a pretty difficult thing to accept – particularly when you may feel guilty already. Many rude people think that it is acceptable to mutter comments under their breath when they see you with your child, or shake their heads in disgust. You may be tempted to offer a raft of excuses, or to lose your temper. Don't. People can be ignorant and rude, and the best thing you can do is to hold your head high and to know that although you might have made mistakes in the past, you are now taking the opportunity to rectify them. If people are ill-mannered or unkind in front of your child, simply point out to your child that only unhappy people feel the need to bully and be unkind to others. Reassure your child that being overweight does not make them a bad or unattractive person, and that what other people think – particularly those that don't even know them – is irrelevant. Such behaviour from others can be a real setback for an emotionally fragile child, and you may have to do a little extra work to make them feel more confident again.

Guilt won't help your child to regain a healthy weight, nor will it be enough to drive you to make changes. Guilt is a negative emotion and it's important to remember that you are making positive changes for positive reasons. You have a game plan and you are going to follow it. What happened in the past is gone. It's time to clear up the damage and move on. Guilt will not change the fact that your child is overweight, nor will it help him to stabilize his weight, but it can make you all feel miserable. Let it go and focus on a more positive future. Take pride in the fact that you have opened your eyes to the reality of the situation and are now doing something about it. It takes great strength to admit a problem and to go about changing the causative factors. You found that strength, so there is no point in holding on to guilt.

What if there's more behind your child's weight gain?

As I pointed out in Chapter 2 there are some children who suffer from other problems that can exacerbate or cause weight gain. If you find that the measures outlined in this book don't seem to be having much effect, it's worth considering the other possible causes. Let's look at some of the things that you can do to make adjustments.

Nutritional deficiencies

Sometimes even a minor deficiency in key vitamins and minerals can cause your child to suffer from cravings, moodiness or health problems that affect his weight – and his ability to lose or stabilize his weight. This is often the case in children who have had a very poor or limited diet – or have relied too heavily on junk foods and fizzy drinks, which tend to rob the body of important nutrients. While a good healthy diet will eventually right any deficiencies, it's worth considering some supplements to kickstart the process. A good multivitamin and mineral tablet should do the trick, taken once or twice a day, with a meal. Make sure it has the following nutrients (a good quality product will list what's included):

Chromium: This mineral is responsible for the GTF (glucose tolerance factor) in our bodies and it reduces sugar cravings. Chromium also helps to control levels of fat and cholesterol in the blood. One study showed that people who took chromium picolinate over a one-week period lost an average of about 2 kg (4.5 lb) of fat more than those taking a placebo (dummy or sugar tablet). Obviously weight loss is not the goal in children, but if your child is deficient in chromium (very common, as it is found naturally in wholegrains, liver, mushrooms and brewer's yeast, which are not high in children's diets) it may be affecting his weight and his ability to sustain normal blood sugar levels.

B vitamins: These have been linked with the improved function of the thyroid gland and fat metabolism. Transporting glucose from the blood into the cells depends on the presence of vitamins B3 (niacin) and B6, and the minerals chromium and zinc.

Vitamin C: Necessary for the normal functioning of your child's glands, vitamin C can also speed up a slow metabolism, prompting it to burn more calories. If your child eats no fruit or vegetables, or very few, he won't be getting enough vitamin C.

Zinc: This is a key mineral in appetite control. It also plays a role, together with vitamins A and E, in the manufacture of the thyroid hormone, which helps to govern energy levels and metabolism.

Calcium: This is involved in the activation of something called 'lipase', an enzyme that breaks down fat for the body to use. Research from Purdue University in Indiana, USA, reveals that a high consumption of calcium slows weight gain. These findings confirm that calcium not only helps to keep weight in check, but can be associated with decreases in body fat. Many kids are calcium deficient, having given up milk in favour of fizzy drinks, or been weaned off dairy produce in an attempt to curb weight gain.

Remember, any imbalances can cause changes in the body which lead to less energy and a greater disposition to laying down fat. If your child has had a poor diet over the years, chances are he will be deficient in a number of key nutrients. A good multi should make all the difference.

One other supplement worth taking is acidophilus and other healthy bacteria, known as 'probiotics'. These help to enhance digestion, which means that nutrients are better absorbed and waste more efficiently eliminated. A sluggish metabolism is often the result of inadequate digestion (and inadequate exercise!) and getting it moving can have a positive effect on weight.

Blood sugar problems

Closely linked to obesity and a whole host of other health and emotional problems is the issue of blood sugar imbalance. And this is a big problem for many kids today, largely because their diets are so high in sugar and refined carbohydrates. We talked about the causes and impact of blood sugar problems in Chapter 3, and the importance of encouraging kids to eat foods that have a lower glycaemic index, in order to keep blood sugar levels stable. But what else can you do?

Obviously it's vital to know if blood sugar is at the root of your child's problem. The following quiz should offer some valuable clues.

Quiz

Answer the following questions:

1 Is your child often tired or unable to concentrate in the afternoon and seems to flag?
2 Does your child's energy go up and down throughout the day, with extreme highs and lows?
3 Does he seem to have more energy after meals – even to the point of seeming a bit hyperactive?

4 Does your child seem groggy in the morning, even if he has slept for the number of hours recommended for his age (see page 165)?
5 Does your child waken in the night feeling anxious?
6 Does your child seem to crave carbohydrates and sweets?
7 Is your child moody? And particularly so if he misses a meal?
8 Is your child irritable in the morning?
9 Is there a history of type 2 diabetes in your family?
10 Does your child seem to be a bit wild after eating small quantities of sugar or sweets?

Interpreting the result

If you have more yes answers than no, there's a possibility that your child has a blood sugar imbalance. If all of your answers are yes, or predominantly yes, talk to your doctor about the possibility of having a specialist check how your child's body deals with sugar. Blood sugar problems can occasionally be an early sign of diabetes.

But remember, even minor blood sugar imbalances can play havoc with your child's moods, his ability to concentrate, his weight, his sleep patterns and his energy levels.

How to deal with blood sugar problems

• Switch to low GI foods whenever possible, and try to ensure that carbohydrates (particularly those with a high GI) are eaten with protein (see page 84).

• Ensure regular meals and snacks to keep levels steady. Breakfast is particularly important (see page 101) and a mid-afternoon snack may be necessary to prevent a slump that will affect energy and concentration.

• Offer small, low-GI snacks mid-afternoon or in advance of a longer stretch without food. It can help nip the problem in the bud.

• Offer a snack before bedtime – some low-GI fruit or a few nuts, or even a piece of wholemeal toast with peanut butter – to prevent the surge of adrenalin which can disrupt sleep.

- Avoid caffeine (in tea, coffee, fizzy drinks and chocolate). Caffeine stimulates the secretion of insulin, effectively destabilizing the blood sugar system. Caffeine, because it has stimulant effects in the body, will almost certainly pick up flagging energy levels, but its effect on blood sugar generally leads to a slump in energy later on. Another downside to caffeine is that it appears to worsen the symptoms of hypoglycaemia.

- Avoid artificial sweeteners. These do not do anything to keep blood sugar levels stable, and are believed to be seriously detrimental to health.

- Make sure your child gets a good multivitamin and mineral tablet that contains chromium, which helps to regulate blood sugar levels and can be effective in combating hypoglycaemia; manganese, which plays an important part in activating the enzymes that are involved in sugar metabolism in the body; magnesium, which is important for blood sugar regulation, and improves the action of insulin; and vitamins B1, B2 and B3, which have a critical role to play in the metabolism of carbohydrate sources of energy in the body. This will help ensure your child's body is balanced and working efficiently.

Food sensitivities

In Chapter 2 we touched upon the subject of food sensitivities and the possibility that they might be at the root of your child's overweight, and it's worth considering this further as a possible factor. Sensitivities are not allergies because they don't involve an allergic reaction, but they do cause the body to react. One of the main symptoms is feeling lethargic and tired after meals, and experiencing a feeling of being not quite well. Other symptoms may include colic, glue ear, ear infections, eczema, asthma or recurrent tonsillitis, excess mucus or catarrh formation, cravings (particularly for things such as bread and cheese), dark circles under the eyes, fluid retention, irritable bowel syndrome (IBS), hives or an undiagnosed rash, abdominal bloating and recurrent, unexplained symptoms.

Most children who are food sensitive have problems with between one and five foods, although older children whose sensitivities have gone undiagnosed for many years may be sensitive or intolerant to many more. Kids may also be sensitive to ingredients in a particular food, or something used in its processing, rather than the food itself, which makes it even harder to work out what is responsible.

Experts suggest that randomly withdrawing foods from a child's diet can be dangerous, leaving it unbalanced at a time when nutrients are required most. If you suspect a food sensitivity, keep a food diary for a week or two. Writing down everything your child eats and their reactions can help you pinpoint foods that might be causing health problems. Sometimes a child will react to food immediately; sometimes within 48 hours, so keep an eye on any response that seems unusual. Many parents have a pretty good idea of foods that might be the culprit, so focus on those first. Wheat and wheat products are a common cause of sensitivities so you may want to keep a close eye on your child's reaction to these. If there doesn't seem to be a problem with wheat, see how he responds to dairy products – another common cause of sensitivities.

If your child shows a reaction to a food, such as being tired, hyperactive, moody or developing a rash, drop it completely for a couple of weeks. However, you must take care to replace it in the diet with a food or group of foods with a similar nutrient content. For example, if you drop wheat or other gluten-containing foods, you must ensure that your child has another source of good-quality unrefined carbohydrates, as well as B vitamins. If you cut out milk and milk products, for example, make sure your child is getting enough protein and calcium from other sources (plenty of green vegetables and pulses, for example). Note, however, that elimination diets are only appropriate for children over the age of five, and that you should never remove more than one food (or food group, as in the case of dairy products for example) at a time. It is beyond the scope of this book to go into food sensitivities in great detail, so if you are unsure, it's definitely worth talking to your doctor before making changes. Broad-scale elimination diets, where many foods are removed at the same time, are not appropriate for children.

A very basic, gentle elimination diet – where one food is removed at a time – should have a fairly immediate effect, and you should notice that the symptoms are alleviated within a few days. After a couple of weeks, reintroduce that food on its own so that any reaction can be assessed. The reaction time after a period of elimination is normally much faster than it would have been when the food was a regular part of the diet. In some children, there is an almost immediate reaction – sneezing, vomiting, hyperactivity or flushing, for example.

A sensitivity to a particular food need not be long term – in many cases children can go on to eat the particular food at a later stage. This usually occurs because they have outgrown their sensitivity, or a break from the foods has allowed their body to adjust. However, it is important that you offer problem foods only occasionally and avoid overindulgence, which may cause the problem to return. You may find that your child becomes sensitive again after an illness or course of antibiotics, or when they are simply run down and tired. In these situations, withdraw the offending food or foods for a week or so and then try them again later. For more information on this complex topic I recommend that you read *The Complete Guide to Food Allergy and Intolerance*, by Dr Jonathan Brostoff and Linda Gamlin (Bloomsbury), or visit www.allergies.about.com, which is an excellent source of information for parents.

What else can you do?

- Encourage your child to chew food thoroughly, as this is essential for proper digestion.

- Avoid big meals, as these increase pressure on the digestive system.

- Avoid offering drinks with meals. Diluted fruit juice or water can be offered before or after meals.

- Many cases of food sensitivities have to do with digestive problems, and the gut itself. Sometimes healing the gut can make a big difference. Giving your child probiotics, which are healthy bacteria, in supplement form is one good way to go about this.

- Ensure that your child's multivitamin and mineral tablet contains at least the recommended daily allowance of vitamins E and A, both of which play an important role in healing the gut lining. In many cases of food allergy, a 'leaky gut' may be at the root of the problem, so ensuring the health of your child's digestive system should help.

Carbohydrate cravings

If your child craves carbohydrates, it will become fairly obvious, fairly instantly. When you start to reduce her intake of unhealthy carbs, she'll have an intense desire for things like sweets, chocolate, white bread and other refined products such as biscuits, crisps, cakes and sugary drinks. Her choice of snacks will be a good indication of this problem.

Research has found that an amino acid, tryptophan, increases in the blood when carbohydrates are eaten. Carbohydrates stimulate the secretion of insulin, which speeds the uptake of tryptophan into the central nervous system where it is converted into serotonin in the brain. Serotonin, in turn, regulates mood and sleepiness. Patients with carbohydrate craving are thought to have a faulty serotonin feedback mechanism that neglects to tell the body to stop craving carbohydrates. When the feedback mechanism is disturbed, the brain fails to respond when carbohydrates are eaten and the desire for them persists.

What can you do?

- Choose carbohydrates that raise the blood sugar slowly (see Low GI foods, page 84), and try to mix them with proteins. For example, eating a biscuit with cheese will ensure the carbs in the biscuit are absorbed much more slowly into the bloodstream. Furthermore, eating food high in protein is thought to promote feelings of fullness and satisfaction, which is vital to weight control.

- Dietary fibre is another useful tool, as it slows the entry of glucose into the bloodstream, reducing spikes in blood sugar levels. This reduction in blood sugar level lowers the amount of insulin production, therefore lowering the amount of glucose that will be stored as fat, reducing cravings and increasing the feeling of fullness. Good sources of fibre are whole, fresh foods, such as whole grains and cereals and fruits and vegetables (raw if possible). Ensure that your child gets plenty of these every day, plus lots of water to ensure that the fibre passes smoothly through her digestive system.

- If cravings seem to strike at the same time every day, interrupt that craving by offering a healthy, low-carbohydrate snack 30 minutes before the craving arrives.

- Limit fruit juices between meals, which can cause a burst of energy, followed by a crash. This will leave your child starved of energy, and produce the craving for high-carbohydrate foods. Caffeine has much the same effect, so cut out anything containing it.

- And remove temptation – staying away from foods high in carbohydrates will be easier if they are not easily accessible.

Depression

Depression is a prolonged feeling of unhappiness and despondency, often magnified by a major life event such as bereavement or parental divorce. Many children and adolescents suffer from depression, which can also be the result of fluctuating hormones or undue stress. It can also follow a viral illness such as glandular fever. There is a strong link between depression and overweight, and if your child appears to have several of the common symptoms, it's worth considering this as a cause.

If your child is depressed, bear in mind that it is an illness and they won't just 'snap out of it'. It's important to be patient and to spend as much time as you can boosting self-esteem (see page 181), even in the depths of despair.

We looked at the large number of possible symptoms of depression in Chapter 2 but here is a quick reminder of some of the common signs to watch out for:

- Becoming withdrawn – avoiding friends, family and regular activities
- Feeling guilty or bad, being self-critical and self-blaming
- Feeling unhappy, miserable and lonely a lot of the time
- Feeling hopeless and wanting to die
- Difficulty in concentrating
- Not looking after your personal appearance
- Difficulty getting off to sleep or waking very early
- Tiredness and lack of energy
- Frequent minor health problems such as headaches or stomach aches.

What can you do?

- Try to remove some of the pressure weighing on your child and create opportunities for him to find activities he enjoys and feels good about doing. A child doesn't have to be wildly popular to be happy, but he does need at least one good friend. Parents also should encourage their child to be active; going to a film or playing ball is more likely to make a child feel better than staying home alone.

- Encourage exercise, which improves mood and encourages the release of endorphins, the 'feel-good' hormones.

- Conversation and communication are extremely important. Practise 'active listening', which basically involves expressing an interest in what your child is doing; and validate his feelings rather than glossing over them or making them seem unimportant.

- Talk to your child's teacher to work out if there is anything at school that could be causing distress or unhappiness. Some schools now offer 'nurturing programmes', where they set up groups to discuss inappropriate behaviour, what hurts, and how to cooperate with one another – with a view to tapping into emotional problems and getting them out in the open. There may be something like that at your child's school. Investigate.

• Offer unconditional love and concern.

• Take time to listen when they want to talk about their feelings.

• Show them you are available without being 'pushy'.

• Encourage them to do things you know they enjoy.

• Notice the little things they are doing that you approve of.

• Support and encourage your child to get help without nagging.

• If your child won't go for help and you are worried, visit your child's doctor yourself. They'll be able to advise you on how to best handle the situation.

Professional help

If you are very worried about your overweight child and he does not seem to respond to any changes to his lifestyle or diet, it's time to consider some extra help. There is no shame in seeking out support from doctors, nurses, counsellors or other specialists, many of whom are trained to deal specifically with the problem of childhood obesity. Sometimes problems escalate beyond the control of parents – and their ability to help.

The first thing to remember when you go for extra help is that any expert you see, or are recommended to see, must be registered and appropriately qualified. Anyone who offers a quick-fix solution, a miracle 'cure' or instant weight loss is either taking advantage of the situation, or potentially dangerous. There are no overnight solutions to weight problems, and they must be dealt with sensitively, and over the long term, by qualified professionals.

Your first port of call should always be your family doctor, who can assess the problem and recommend the appropriate specialists, should they be necessary. He might recommend a dietitian, or a visit to a specially qualified nurse. He may also suggest counselling, or behaviour modification (see below), to get to grips with a problem that has an emotional basis. Some doctors can also recommend 'fat camps' or other facilities where kids will be taught about nutrition and exercise – and encouraged to take part in activities – under the guidance of trained professionals, and in the company of other children in the same boat. This can sometimes be a good plan for a child who is at his wits' end, and really wants to do something about his weight without feeling different or embarrassed in front of lighter peers. But before you undertake anything like this, make sure you and your doctor talk it through with your child, and only go through with it if your child is motivated and agrees to give it a try. It may be that you have to try a few sessions together, to see if you child feels comfortable. If it's not right for your child, don't push it.

Exercise specialists can also be recommended, to help develop a programme for a child that takes into consideration his particular

BEHAVIOUR MODIFICATION

This is a set of techniques aimed at addressing specific behavioural problems in pre-teenagers and adolescents. It comprises a number of therapeutic intervention techniques designed to give the child tools to change their negative behaviours. The techniques tend to be highly effective in children and teenagers, primarily because unlike adults, they are not set in their ways. The younger a child is, the more effective behaviour modification techniques can be.

Behaviour modification focuses on increasing motivation to change diet and physical activity level, using a combination of short-term individual and family psychotherapy sessions. Sessions are based on literally modifying your child's behaviour so she'll learn better ways to cope with stress, depression or unhappiness; how to recognize cues that make her want to eat or overeat; and strategies for dealing with environmental factors that affect her eating habits. For example, eating in one room of the house only, or avoiding the route home that goes past all the food shops. She'll also learn how to take a more positive direction in terms of lifestyle – watching less TV and spending less time being sedentary.

Studies show that in combination with a healthy diet and a more active lifestyle, behaviour modification can be hugely effective.

CASE HISTORY: # Tom

Tom's dad was the main cook in their household, and got great pleasure from feeding up his 'big lad'. A full cooked breakfast started his day every morning, and there was never any shortage of snacks available at home. Indeed, Tom's 'normal' after-school snack was some frozen pizza or a couple of microwaved burgers. Tom had always been tall for his age, and fairly active, but when he hit his teenage years, he began to take more interest in computers, which meant long hours in front of a screen. His growth settled down at this time and, not surprisingly, he put on a great deal of weight across a short period of time – although at 15 he was 1.8 m (nearly 6 ft) tall, he also weighed well in excess of 113 kg (250 lb). He voluntarily went to see the family doctor, who suggested a summer 'fat camp', which ran for four weeks every summer across the holiday season. The camp was designed for kids who were seriously overweight and they were given lots of incentive to exercise and plenty of healthy food to choose from. Tom attended the camp for three years running, each time

losing a substantial amount of weight. He always came away with good intentions but over the school year his old habits returned and he began a bit of a yo-yo cycle of weight loss and weight gain, which left him frustrated and demoralized.

Tom was eventually referred to a counsellor, who specialized in behaviour modification. She was able to teach Tom to identify the factors that caused him to overeat; one of which was the joy he got from pleasing his dad by eating whatever he cooked. His whole family then became involved in the 'change', and the cupboards were restocked with healthier options – out went the frozen pizzas, the deep-fried goodies, the microwaved meals that were Tom's 'snacks'. His dad agreed to start running with him in the mornings – to share time together that did not involve food. Over the course of a year, Tom's weight stabilized, and he grew to his full height of 1.88 m (6 ft 2 in). He also established a healthier relationship with his dad who also, interestingly, lost over 19 kg (3 stone) in the process.

needs and overall level of fitness. If you are offered this opportunity, grab it. Your child will get plenty of attention, and lots of ideas to inspire him to develop healthy exercise habits.

If your child's weight loss is related to hormones or growth, you may be referred to an endocrinologist – basically a hormone specialist – who can run tests and provide details of an appropriate diet and/or medication.

To locate a weight-control programme for your child, you may wish to contact your local hospital, university or college. There may even be an obesity clinic at your doctor's surgery, which offers a good, well-rounded programme. The overall goal of a treatment programme should be to help your whole family adopt healthy eating and physical activity habits that you can keep up for the rest of your lives. Here are some other things a weight-control programme should do:

• Include a variety of health care professionals on staff: doctors, dietitians, psychiatrists or psychologists, and/or exercise physiologists.

• Evaluate your child's weight, growth and health before they enrol in the programme and monitor their progress throughout.

• Adapt to the specific age and abilities of your child. Programmes for four-year-olds should be different from those for 12-year-olds.

• Help your family keep up healthy eating and physical activity behaviours after the programme ends.

• Include a maintenance programme and other support and referral resources to reinforce the new behaviours and to deal with underlying issues that contributed to overweight.

In the Resources section you will find lots of sources of information and help for you and your overweight child.

Drugs and surgery

There are prescription-only drugs available to help very obese people to lose weight. These are not, however, miracle drugs and many have serious side-effects. There are very few instances where drugs will be recommended for children, and I suggest you think very carefully about agreeing to any drug that claims to promote weight loss. The idea is that children should grow into their weight, rather than attempt to actively lose it. And even though weight-loss drugs are only prescribed for a one-year period, they are not suitable for growing, developing children.

You may be offered drugs to treat hormonal disorders or other health or emotional conditions underlying your child's weight problem. Ask about the side-effects – and if there are any other options – before considering this type of treatment. A good consultant will be able to supply you with all the information you need.

There are several types of surgery for very obese adults, which are normally used as a last resort. These are not, under any circumstances, appropriate for children.

In conclusion

Don't be embarrassed about asking for help and enlisting support. It's a difficult job being a parent at the best of times. There are many specialists who can help if you run into trouble, or have concerns that don't appear to be addressed by changing your child's diet and lifestyle. There will always be periods, too, when you feel out of your depth and don't know where to turn. In the next chapter we'll look at some of the most common problems associated with helping an overweight child, and the best ways to deal with them as and when they occur.

Chapter Eight

Troubleshooting

This chapter is designed to help you to deal with various problems that crop up as you take steps to help your overweight child. Even the healthiest, happiest children suffer problems and setbacks from time to time, and it would be idealistic to think that making changes will mean plain sailing from here on in. Use this chapter as quick reference when you come across a specific problem or issue, or if you have a question that doesn't seem to be answered in the first part of this book.

Bingeing

If your child is a regular binger, he might have a binge-eating disorder. Binge eating episodes usually involve:

- Eating an unusually large amount of food in a short period of time (within 2 hours)
- A feeling of having no control over eating or the ability to stop eating during the episode.

As well as the above, a binge eater will also exhibit at least three of the following characteristics:

- Eating more quickly than normal
- Eating until feeling uncomfortably full
- Eating large amounts of food when not physically hungry
- Eating alone due to embarrassment over the amount he is eating
- Feeling disgusted with himself, depressed, or very guilty after overeating.

While any bingeing is undoubtedly unhealthy, it becomes a 'disorder' if it occurs at least two days a week for at least six months. Binge eaters have episodes of overeating only – with no regular use of vomiting, fasting, excessive exercise or laxatives to rid themselves of the food. The overeating is not associated with anorexia or bulimia.

It's worth noting that research shows that many overweight and obese children suffer from a binge-eating problem. If you are worried, seek help from your doctor. Many children do need some help from a counsellor or psychologist to overcome the problem. Consider the following:

• In a calm and caring way, tell your child that you are aware of his bingeing. Let him know that you are concerned.

• Make it clear that it is OK to eat when he is hungry, but that overeating will make him ill.

• Listen carefully to what your child says. Children who binge-eat might feel ashamed or afraid. They might feel out of control. You may be able to help them get some control back, by offering to help them the next time they feel an urge to binge.

• It is very common for kids with problems to say that there is nothing wrong. Tell them you want to help. You may need to approach them several times.

• Make sure you don't have unhealthy foods lying around that might tempt your child.

• Make sure he has at least three good meals a day, plus snacks, so that he doesn't feel hungry. Although binge eating usually has nothing to do with hunger, it's less likely to occur in children who feel satisfied.

• Look for emotional causes – problems at school, worries, stress or any other underlying problems. If you can deal with the causative factor, you are halfway to winning the battle.

• Make sure your child doesn't feel ashamed about his size or about eating in general. Many overweight children are so embarrassed about their size, they feel awkward eating anything in public – or in front of the family – for fear of recrimination. Make sure your child is not singled out for special attention in your family, and that he doesn't feel different or 'fat'. If he feels good about himself, he's much less likely to binge for emotional reasons.

• Help your child learn when to stop. Explain that eating when he isn't hungry will only make him feel worse. Keep him active so that he isn't tempted to eat to make up for perceived failures or to deal with problems.

Bullying

This problem seems to be part and parcel of being overweight, and your child may well experience it at some stage, even if it is not full-blown harassment. We outlined the extent of bullying on pages 170–171, and the effect it has on a child's self-esteem. There are, however, things you can do to help:

• If you suspect bullying but your child won't confirm it, look out for clues – for example, mysteriously 'lost' belongings, inexplicable bruises, withdrawn behaviour and mystery ailments that prevent your child from having to go to school. If you are concerned, try to encourage your child to talk about it. Ask about different parts of their day and about the people they like and don't like. Ask if lunchtime or break is stressful and why. Don't bully them into talking, which will just make matters worse. Just let them know that you are there if they want to share the problem.

• Talk to your child's school and find out what anti-bullying policies they have in place. Chances are they don't know what is going on, and they can take steps to stop it.

• It's also important that your child develops her own coping strategies. Suggest some sharp retorts that your child could use, or ways of avoiding the perpetrators. Overweight children tend to have lower self-esteem than their peers, perhaps unconsciously placing themselves in a 'victim' mode. Work on your child's self-esteem (see page 181). If she feels good about herself and confident, she'll be able to face up to bullies and hold her own.

• Make sure she realizes her own worth, and understands that bullies have problems of their own. Give her the higher ground.

• Explain to your child why some people become bullies. Bullies are normally victims of someone else in their lives. If your child is aware that there is a cause for the behaviour unrelated to her, she may feel more in control of the situation.

• Your child does, however, need to learn to stand up for herself with confidence. Practise what she could say to bullies, and help her to feel comfortable remembering and using these words. For example, 'Stop calling me names now, I don't like it and I'm not going to accept it any more'. There's a veiled threat there that further action could be taken, and even the most robust bully fears recrimination from authorities. The secret is for your child to look strong and confident, and to look the bully/ies in the eye while holding up her head.

• Make sure your child doesn't feel guilty, which can compound the problem. Many children blame themselves, and believe that their own weakness or perceived problem led to the bullying. Help them to feel that they are not in any way at fault and that they are good, strong, effective people – even if they are overweight.

• Don't become too upset. It won't help your child, and she may become alarmed, over-sensitive, or concerned that she has made you unhappy. Be calm and supportive, and show her that you are on her side and are prepared to show a little of that all-important family solidarity.

- Some children need an awful lot of comfort alongside the solutions. Don't be too business-like or problem-focused. Ensure you give plenty of hugs, reassurance, love and empathy. Your child will be feeling very vulnerable and may need more love than practical advice.

- Encourage your child to develop friendships outside of school, in sports, musical groups, drama organizations and so on. If she builds up a strong network of friends outside school, who share her interests and enjoy her company, she'll feel stronger and more able to cope with bullies the rest of the time. Ensure that your child does have a good circle of friends at school, and encourage this if possible. Children in a group are much less likely to be bullied than children alone.

Comfort eating

Children often eat to fill the emptiness they feel on the inside (as do adults). Overeating is often considered an eating disorder. At the core of an eating disorder lies the need for the child or the adolescent to have control. How will the overweight children take control? Eat more, of course! It's not surprising that kids turn to food for comfort. Parents often unwittingly encourage this when their children are young – offering a treat when they have hurt themselves, or when they are upset, lonely or down for any reason. Kids then develop an association between food and feeling good.

As kids get older, too, food can become a 'friend'. It makes them feel good, fills them up and makes no demands of them. And when kids become seriously overweight, they can become very isolated, which compounds the problem. So what can you do?

- If you notice your child eating large quantities of food after school and heading for the computer or TV, sit down next to them and ask, 'How was your day?' Don't let them eat to make themselves feel better. Let them talk to you about their problems.

- Your reaction to your child's weight can be more devastating than the actual excess pounds. When parents put pressure on children to lose weight, children often feel like a failure if they don't. Children cannot be expected to make changes on their own – the whole family has to change its lifestyle. Don't single out the overweight child by making one special meal for them, instead get the whole family to eat well.

- Older children can be taught to understand the reasons why they overeat for comfort – and learn to make associations between triggers and overeating. Suggest that your child keeps a food diary. Ask her to keep track of how she is feeling when she eats at different points of the day. She may find that she eats after school, when she is feeling low, or that she eats when she is bored or lonely. She may even choose food for solace when she is angry or upset. Go through her diary with her, and help her to see where the problem areas are. Teach her different ways to cope (see Chapter 6 page 192), and suggest that every time she feels the need to eat to fill an emotional requirement, she could take some exercise instead, or come and talk to you, or even learn a form of relaxation, such as yoga.

- Make sure you stop using food as a pick-me-up for your child. A trip to the cinema, a walk together or a new book are much healthier 'treats' to lift spirits.

- Not all children eat for emotional reasons. Some children eat because they are bored. In this case, you'll need to ensure that your child has a busier schedule, activities to choose from, and friends to see. If she doesn't have a circle of friends, try to enrol her in a class or activity where she will meet some.

- Show some self-restraint yourself. If you reach for the chocolates or a glass of wine when you are stressed or upset, you are teaching the wrong behaviours.

Cravings

See Chapter 7 page 215

Eating disorders

One of the problems with overweight is that it can, in extreme circumstances, lead to eating disorders. Children who struggle with their weight look for quick-fix solutions, and can develop very unhealthy relationships with food. Not all overweight kids develop eating disorders, particularly if the problem is addressed as early as possible, nor do many children with eating disorders even have a problem with weight. In fact, in many cases, they are a perfectly healthy weight, but they perceive themselves to be fat. This is one reason why it is important to deal with issues relating to food and weight at a very early age. Children need to feel good about themselves, and to have a positive body image.

It's beyond the scope of this book to go into the problems associated with eating disorders in any detail, but it's worth looking out for a few key pointers that a problem might be on its way – or already an issue. You will also find the details of organizations that can help on page 252 of the Resources section.

Anorexia nervosa

While it may seem odd to feature anorexia in a book on overweight children, it's important to be aware that if a child has suffered abuse for being 'fat', they may consider themselves to be fat and unattractive long after the weight has shifted, and this could influence their future behaviour. A poor self-image is almost always at the root of an eating disorder but the media and its emphasis on super-thin models is also blamed by some for influencing the way people, particularly girls, see themselves and for encouraging them to believe that looks are all-important.

According to the Eating Disorders Association in the UK, girls as young as five are reported to be weight-conscious, and thinking about dieting. In the US, over 60 per cent of fourth grade girls (about nine years old) in an Iowa study reported a desire to be thinner. By age 18, nine out of 10 teenage girls in a Californian survey were dieting to lose weight.

Anorexia nervosa is a form of intentional self-starvation. What may begin as a normal diet is carried to extremes, with many reducing their intake to an absolute minimum.

The average age for onset of the illness is thought to be 16, although the age range of anorexia is between 10 and 40. Around 90 per cent of sufferers are female. While most sufferers have no history of being overweight, it is prudent – particularly if you have a teenage daughter – to be aware of this devastating condition.

Warning signs

• Does your child seem obsessed by fat or the calorie content of food? Has she put herself on a 'diet' for any reason, and cannot be swayed from it?

• Does your child exercise obsessively, carefully calculating the number of calories burned during physical activity?

• Is your child frequently 'not hungry' or 'too busy' at mealtimes?

• Does your child disappear into the lavatory after meals?

• Have you noticed any mood changes, including angry outbursts, isolation from friends, withdrawn behaviour, chemical abuse or depression. Studies indicate that starvation tends to increase feelings of depression, anxiety, irritability and anger, and mood is a good sign that all is not well. Beware, however, many teens are subject to mood swings, so if this is the only symptom, look elsewhere for a cause.

• Has your daughter failed to start her period at a normal time, or has it stopped?

• Apart from weight loss, does your child suffer from dry skin, hair loss, rashes and itching?

Bulimia nervosa

Bulimia is thought to be two to three times more common than anorexia, but is not generally as physically dangerous. However, excessive use of laxatives and self-induced vomiting can cause rupture of the oesophagus, mineral deficiency and dehydration, which can have serious effects on health.

Bulimia was only officially recognized in the 1970s and is characterized by a cycle of bingeing and starving. Many bulimics seem fine, but experts say that, under the surface, they often suffer from poor self-esteem and self-image. Bulimics may have irregular periods or stop having periods at all because of excessive use of laxatives and vomiting. Using laxatives can also cause kidney and bowel problems and stomach disorders.

Warning signs

It can be more difficult to recognize this condition, because your child may stay around the same weight, or lose weight more slowly. Look out for the following:

Psychological signs
- Uncontrollable urges to eat vast amounts of food
- An obsession with food, or feeling 'out of control' around food
- Distorted perception of body weight and shape
- Emotional behaviour and mood swings
- Anxiety and depression; low self-esteem, shame and guilt
- Isolation – feeling helpless and lonely

Behavioural signs
- Bingeing and vomiting
- Disappearing to the toilet after meals in order to vomit food eaten
- Excessive use of laxatives, diuretics or enemas
- Periods of fasting
- Excessive exercise
- Secrecy and reluctance to socialize
- Shoplifting for food; abnormal amounts of money spent on food
- Food disappearing unexpectedly or being secretly hoarded

Some experts believe bulimia is the result of an imbalance of chemicals in the brain, but others think the illness is more likely to be linked to a lack of self-worth. It is thought that up to half of anorexics also suffer from bulimia and some 40 per cent of bulimics are reported to have a history of anorexia.

Preventing eating disorders

• Children who are anorexic are much more likely to be a product of a family who are over-concerned about weight and diet (and, for example, the fat content of food). Avoid talking about weight or diets, even though your child does have a weight problem. Parents send strong messages to their children when they constantly complain about their bodies, discuss diets and obsess over the fat, calorie and sugar content of food.

• Make family meals a daily occurrence. Do not reach the stage where you have not eaten with your children, or seen them eating, for weeks – and certainly not months. Children should *not* be made responsible for their own food choices. Apart from the fact that they can easily make unacceptable choices that can damage their health, parents need to model positive eating habits, which will go a long way towards instilling healthy attitudes to food and eating.

• Always provide a variety of fresh foods from all food groups at meals. Don't force a child to eat, and give small helpings. They can always ask for more.

• Parents have a powerful influence on their children's self-esteem and body image. In one study, the self-esteem scores of kids aged nine to 11 were lowered when they thought their parents were dissatisfied with their bodies. Encourage your child to feel good about himself, no matter what his weight. Even if he is very fat, he needs high self-esteem (see page 181). Make sure your child feels loved and accepted for what he is, not what he looks like. Children with high self-esteem naturally gravitate towards habits that are good for them – taking exercise, having good hygiene habits, dressing well and taking pride in their appearance (flaws and all!).

What to do if your child suffers from an eating disorder

• You will need to tackle emotional issues in order to uncover what is affecting their self-image and self-esteem (see page 181). The most important thing you can do is support and love your child. Showing disgust when he is overly thin or fat will reinforce a poor self-image. Let your child know that you love him and care about him. You can certainly show concern about his health, but make sure he is aware that your love and concern are not judgmental.

• Encourage hobbies and activities that will help your child to feel good about himself – choose something at which he is bound to succeed. Draw attention to successes and overlook failures of any kind.

• Get some help for yourself. Contact a support group (see Resources page 251). Try not to blame yourself. There is a great deal of finger-pointing going on about eating disorders, and parents often take full brunt. Even secure children can suffer from self-esteem and emotional problems after an upset, or there may be problems at school that you know nothing about. The best advice is to get to the root of the problem, and to find ways of addressing it. A good port of call for advice is the Eating Disorders Association (see page 252).

Embarrassment

Overweight children who are conscious of their problem often feel embarrassed and ashamed of their size, and go to great lengths to avoid interaction with others, exercise (which can be hugely awkward) and even eating in public. The taunting that they may have experienced will have compounded the problem, and they may experience extremely low self-esteem as a result.

As dreadful as it may be to witness your child suffering in this way, you can't live your child's life for them. They need to learn to be resilient, and to take charge as a way of coping with their overweight. In other words, while you should always show sympathy and understanding, it's also very important to provide your child with the tools he needs to make changes. All of the suggestions in this book are relevant to helping your overweight child regain both a healthy weight and a healthy level of self-esteem. If you explain to your child that being proactive, and making changes, will be a positive first step to overcoming the problem, you should be able to inspire him to do something about it. If he is embarrassed about his weight, there are a number of things you can do to ease this.

Firstly, it's very important that you don't put your child in a position of feeling greater embarrassment when you work on increasing activity levels or changing his diet. He won't want to feel different and he won't want to stand out. He will also want to avoid the ignominy of being the only fat and unfit kid at the fitness centre, so make sure you find appropriate activities for him to begin with (see pages 154–158).

The most important thing you can do, however, is to improve your child's self-esteem, so that he feels good about himself, no matter what his size. There are plenty of overweight adults and children who have a strong, healthy self-image. Your child can be one of them. He needs to learn that being overweight is a temporary problem that he has the resources to address. Just like other kids have asthma, or eczema or skin problems, he has a health issue that needs to be treated. The good news is that unlike some health conditions, his problem is treatable. Inspire him. Fill him with hope. Lift his self-esteem, and let him see that he has no need to be embarrassed about being himself – that he is worthy in his own right, no matter how much he weighs. (See pages 181–187 for more on raising children's self-esteem.)

Faddy eating

See Chapter 4 page 118.

Fad diets

From time to time, your child will be tempted to try fad diets as a quick-fix solution. She may have seen you try various diets yourself, and think that it's better to shift pounds rather than wait until she grows into them. Discourage this at all costs. Fad diets deprive the body of valuable nutrients that your child needs to grow, develop and learn, and they teach her nothing about the healthy eating habit that she will need to carry into adulthood. Show her the statistics: diets *do not* work (see pages 36–39), and they can make over-weight problems worse. Furthermore, children who begin the fad diet rollercoaster tend to be at greater risk of eating disorders. Show her the correct way to lose or stabilize weight – by being more active and eating well. She didn't become overweight overnight, and she won't be come thin overnight.

Peer pressure

Children rate their peers highly, and their status among their peer groups will always be an issue. A recent study showed that most children spent time with their friends either every day or most days (61 per cent) and over two-thirds felt they had extensive friendship networks (68 per cent). This type of peer relationship is healthy and normal. But in an overweight child, peers can represent something different – first of all, they may feel huge pressure to look the same, when they clearly do not, which adds to the problem of low self-esteem. No child wants to feel different. Secondly, many children's attempts to control their weight through healthy eating are under-mined by peer pressure – again, they want to eat the same things that their friends do and they also don't want to be embarrassed by having to make different choices. Thirdly, many overweight kids do not have large circles of friends, mainly because they do not have the self-confidence or self-esteem to make and maintain friendships.

Peer pressure only really becomes a problem when your child is forced into situations in which he feels uncomfortable. By the nature of the term, there will always be 'pressure', but that pressure can be stimulating rather than stifling or frightening. The key is self-esteem. Your child has to respect and believe in himself, and he has to feel confident in his own skin. He needs the courage to stand up for himself, and to challenge his peers when he feels threatened or uncomfortable.

All children should have a hidden reservoir of self-esteem and self-confidence. Reinforce this quality in your children, and teach them to be independent. Give them some power in their household, so that they are used to exerting some control over their environment. If they feel pressured, ask them why someone else's beliefs should be more important than their own, and ask them to challenge or question friends who put them under pressure. Teach him a 'who cares' approach to pressure. In the end, who cares whether you eat fast food or don't? Why should it bother your friends? Who cares if you aren't exactly like your friends. You are unique and wonderful. Celebrate your child's uniqueness rather than struggling to help him to conform. You'll encourage an independence of mind and spirit that will help him through all types of pressure in life.

Be available for communication, and to talk things through. If your child can express his concerns, and get your support at home, he'll feel stronger and more able to cope outside the home environment. It may sound trite, but if you teach your child to believe in himself and his achievements, he will be much more likely to resist external influences and feel comfortable doing so. Point out the importance of true friendship. If he's fallen in with a bunch of people who scorn him, or put him under pressure to conform, it may be time to find new friends.

Ultimately, however, help your child to foster friendships and relationships that are stimulating and non-threatening. If he has a circle of friends around him who support rather than undermine his confidence, he's much less likely to be pressured into doing things that he doesn't want to do. And he's much more likely to develop interests that take the pressure off his situation. If he's out and about, he's less likely to be focusing on food, or feeling low and under-confident. Encourage plenty of activities that involve a wide variety of different children. If he has some recourse or respite from a peer group that is causing or creating too much pressure, he can escape to another and let off a little steam.

It's also important to remember that peer pressure can be positive. The peer group can be a source of affection, sympathy and understanding, particularly when the people in it have the same outlook and are experiencing the very same emotions and situations. That's one reason why you should encourage friendships and activities in your overweight child – and if he is very overweight, he may find comfort in the company of other kids who are in the same boat. Kids need to feel like they belong, and that they have shared interests and problems. Peers can be an important safety net.

Be understanding and empathetic about problems that develop with peers. It's often difficult to relate to what our children are experiencing, particularly if we don't like the company they are keeping, but if we keep the channels of communication open, our children can use us as sounding boards and as a kind of moral linchpin, which gives them a feeling of security. Children also need to know that peer groups are not stable; they should expect to change groups of friends as a part of normal behaviour and growing up. Being aware that they may fall out of favour with peers but will always have the love and acceptance of their family helps ease the blow when they have arguments or 'break-ups'.

Pocket money

Kids need pocket money in order to learn responsibility and, of course, the value of money. They need to be able to learn to budget, and to make sensible choices. It's part of growing up, and one of the first steps towards independence. They need to learn to make their own choices – to see that spending all of their money in one go means that they won't be able to afford that new CD, or go to the cinema with their friends at the weekend. So it's very important that parents do not try to over-control pocket money.

The problem is, of course, that many children blow all of their pocket money on sweets, junk food and fast foods. All of which contribute to a weight problem. Kids who are deprived of goodies at home are even more likely to exhibit this type of behaviour. So while it is important not to intervene too much, it is crucial that you offer some guidance. Reiterate the message about unhealthy eating and what it does to our bodies. Strike a deal – some money can be diverted to the sweet shop, but some must also be put aside or 'saved' and then the remainder can be used for whatever your child wishes. You may find that he uses his money sneakily, and purchases, hides and then eats food when he is alone. If you cotton on to this, do not hesitate to confront him. Make it clear that the family rules are that sweets are allowed for the occasional treat, and certainly not more than once or twice a week. If he wants to buy treats, ask him to put them in the family cupboard, and to eat them in the place of another treat (pudding one night, for example).

You don't have to deny your child the pleasure of spending his money on forbidden goods, because that's something that all children do, regardless of weight. But you do need to lay down some sensible guidelines. The same goes for eating out with friends. Sure, he can use his money for fast food very occasionally, but he must make some sensible choices, too. If he has a burger, he should think about skipping the chips and the fizzy drink. If he has pizza, he needs to go for water on the side and so on. You can use the opportunity to teach your child to make choices about his eating habits – the kind of choices he will need to make throughout his life. Suggest that he spends his money going bowling or swimming some of the time. Try to take the focus away from food, if all of his money is being drained in that direction. Be honest when you talk to your child – don't use subversive methods to influence him, discuss your concerns openly and encourage him to be honest too.

Regression

Sigmund Freud described several mechanisms that children may use to defend themselves against the anxieties or uncertainties of growing up. A child who experiences too much anxiety or too many conflicts at any stage of development may retreat to an earlier, less traumatic stage. Such developmental reversals are examples of a defence mechanism that Freud called 'regression'. Even a well-adjusted adult may regress from time to time in order to forget problems or reduce anxiety, and children, who are less likely to think through and overcome emotional difficulties are even more likely to revert to behaviours that they associate with comfort and care.

This is particularly relevant for overweight children. When under pressure, they revert to earlier, happier times, and many happy memories of childhood involve food. So comfort eating is very often associated with regression. Children may also regress to childlike behaviours – sucking thumbs, or even using baby talk. This is a sign of pressure, and it's important that you find out the cause rather than battling to deal with the symptom. Overweight children face obvious pressures, and it's important to acknowledge them and to teach your child how to cope (see Chapter 6 page 192).

One thing that you can do to address regressive behaviours is to teach children an emotional vocabulary, so that they can verbalize their emotions and literally 'get them off their chest'. Problems that are internalized tend to come out as problem behaviours – such as comfort eating, wetting the bed or resorting to comfort toys. Emotional expression is therefore an incredibly important skill for all children to learn, and one that they will use throughout their lives as they face and learn to cope with stress and anxiety.

Smoking

It can be a considerable obstacle if your child decides that smoking is a quick route to losing weight. A recent study found that it is important for pre-teenagers to have a healthy body image before they hit puberty, in order to reduce the risk that they'll take up smoking as a weight-control measure.

Anne-Luise Winter, a research co-ordinator with the Institute for Clinical Evaluative Sciences, headed a study in which teenage girls who believed they were overweight, or who used even moderate weight control methods, were found more likely to smoke than those who considered themselves average or too thin. Boys who skipped meals to control their weight were also more likely to smoke.

According to Winter, 'By the time puberty starts, they've already heard from their friends all about smoking and weight-control methods and it might be too late to catch it at that time.' However, as she points out, it's not clear whether smoking actually works as a weight-loss measure. Nor has a physiological mechanism for smoking-related weight loss been established. Adult smokers have a lower body mass index than non-smokers, but adolescent smokers tend to weigh more than non-smokers.

Of the students studied, almost one-third (31 per cent) of girls considered themselves overweight, compared to 14 per cent of boys. Girls who believed themselves to be overweight were about 50 per cent more likely to be smokers than those who believed themselves to be of average weight or too thin. Girls were also more likely to smoke if they exercised to lose weight, skipped meals, vomited or used diet pills. Boys who said they skipped meals in order to control their weight were more than twice as likely to smoke as those who did not skip meals.

So what can you do?

The obvious first step is to ensure, as early as possible, that your child has a positive body image (see page 180). You'll also need to make it clear at an early age that smoking is extremely dangerous for health. If you smoke yourself, and also diet, you're setting a very poor example, and that's something that you must address.

If your child does start smoking, and uses weight control as an excuse for continuing, point out the fact that young smokers tend to be more overweight than their non-smoking peers. In other words, it won't work – and they'll damage their health in the process. And hit them with the figures – smoking is still the number one cause of cancer in most parts of the world. However, given that teenagers find it virtually impossible to imagine that they will ever die or become seriously ill, the most effective approach may be to point out the imme-diate unpleasant consequences, like smelly breath and stained fingers, rather than giving them a warning about what may happen in 20 or 30 years!

Addiction to smoking is both physical and psychological. Many smokers find it very difficult to stop smoking and do not succeed. They get physically addicted to the nicotine in cigarettes, which causes real withdrawal symptoms if you cut down or quit. Psychological addiction occurs because smoking becomes a habit. It may help to address the root cause of smoking, such as boredom or insecurity, or a preoccupation with weight.

It's important to make clear the fact that there are no quick-fix solutions to overweight. The single and only way to achieve a bal-anced weight is to become more active, eat healthily, adopt healthy leisure pursuits, and deal with emotional problems in a positive and proactive way. Encourage the teenager to take up sports, for example, and to carry out another activity when they feel the need to have a cigarette. For more information and advice, contact ASH (details on page 257).

Setbacks

There will always be setbacks on the road to a healthier weight. Your child may appear completely in control and flourishing, only to suffer a setback where she begins to crave foods again, or eat for comfort, sneak foods, binge or develop an over-hearty appetite. The most important thing to remember is that your child is not on a diet, and a setback does not mean that anything is ruined. If she falls off the horse, she must be encouraged to get right back on.

If you are careful about ensuring that your child has enough to eat, that she has a reasonable amount of snacks, the odd treat, and isn't going hungry, she is unlikely to feel deprived. If a child is overly restricted, she will develop obsessions about and cravings for food and therefore find any healthy living programme difficult to master. If setbacks are common, you need to consider whether she is getting what she needs.

Furthermore, setbacks do tend to occur when other factors, such as stress, emotional problems or even ill health occur. The natural response in such circumstances is to return to old, comfortable habits, which are easier to live with and instantly satisfying or comforting. In order to overcome these types of setbacks, you need to work out what the cause might be and teach your child to find other ways to cope – more exercise, which raises self-esteem and mood, some time spent with family and friends, or even just a good long talk through any problems she might be experiencing. The sooner she learns to find other ways to cope, the sooner her old habits will disappear for good.

Don't be dispirited by a setback, and don't let your child feel embarrassed or ashamed of reverting to old habits. Explain why she may have drifted or felt the need to escape a little, but help her to see that the changes you have made to your lifestyle will make her feel much better in the long run. Setbacks tend to be short-term problems, and it's important to remind her of this.

In the long term, setbacks simply don't matter. You have changed your way of life, not wed yourself to a strict diet or lifestyle regime. Everyone gives in to treats now and then and occasionally your carefully laid plans will go out the window, usually in times of stress or busy family periods. For long-term changes to be effective, you have to be flexible and realize that life is for living and enjoying – not suffering or deprivation. If your child feels hungry or pressured, you'll never teach the type of habits she needs to acquire for a lifetime of good health and balanced weight. Adjust the programme – her diet and her activities – so that they are better balanced, and there is more time for her, she has more say in what she does, and there are lots of delicious healthy foods on offer to satisfy her appetite. Then carry on.

Sneaking food

Children who sneak food tend to be embarrassed about eating in front of others, or ashamed of the choices they are making. Eating in this way is often the result of cravings (see page 215), or a perceived need for some comfort. The main cause of sneaky eating, however, tends to be an overly restrictive diet. Make sure your child is getting enough to eat, that he has plenty of healthy snacks, and that there are treats occasionally. With peers and the media making clear the message that fast, junk food is fun and 'cool', it's not surprising that kids want foods that they shouldn't eat. Children need to learn why some foods are healthy and why others are not. The unhealthy foods should be eaten only sparingly, and you can come to a compromise about how often that is. Totally denying your child these foods will lead to problems.

You should, however, avoid stocking any foods that you don't want your child to eat. He can't sneak treats from the cupboard if there aren't any. And pocket money can be negotiated and its expenditure agreed (see page 237).

If you find that your child is sneaking food, you should confront him about it. Be patient and understanding, and ask the reasons why he wanted the particular food. Chances are he just wanted a sugar fix, or fancied something that you won't let him have. This is your chance to offer a little education and, again, agree some compromises. Don't make him feel ashamed. You want your child to develop healthy eating habits – and feel comfortable eating in front of others. Make it clear that if he wants an inappropriate snack he should either ask you (if he is young enough to do so) or (if he is older) eat it in front of you. Secret eating is not part of a healthy eating programme.

Stress

Not so long ago, it would have been considered absurd to consider treating a child for stress, but we now know that children are as susceptible to its effects as adults. In some cases it can be worse, because they cannot always verbalize their emotions in the same way that adults can.

Every child is able to cope with a different amount of stress in their lives. Some children happily sail from ballet class to swimming lessons, easily fitting in homework and an exhaustive series of social engagements. Another child would find this lifestyle stressful, and would bow under the pressure. A child who is overweight will have a different set of stresses to children of a healthier weight – peer pressure, bullying, low self-esteem and an overwhelming concern about his weight and how he should deal with it. In periods of stress, many children can regress (see page 238), and seek out comfort foods and even exhibit self-destructive behaviour. They may lose their motivation and feel useless and depressed. Stress is therefore one of the biggest causes of setbacks.

Stress can have many other sources – difficulties at school, exams, too much homework, an over-scheduled life, parental divorce, breaking up with a boyfriend or even insufficient relaxation time – but it can also stem from anything that causes the body to work harder, including a poor diet, inadequate sleep or exercise and even injury.

If you add up the stresses that your child is subject to, you may find that that they are being faced with more than they can easily handle. The numerous possible symptoms of stress are set out in

Chapter 2 (see pages 56–58) but the following symptoms are the most obvious:

• increased breathing and heart rate
• nausea
• tense muscles
• inability to relax
• irritability (including temper tantrums)
• insomnia
• allergies
• skin problems
• headaches
• fatigue
• changes in eating habits

How to help your child

Some stress is healthy and invigorating, but in excess it can cause health to decline on all levels – affecting the function of all systems in the body, including appetite, metabolism and mood. Relaxation is essential. Ensure that your child has time for hobbies that interest him, and which give him satisfaction and pride. The feel-good factor will go a long way towards reducing the effects of stress in other parts of his life.

• Take care that your child isn't overstretched. He might be a determined child who likes to be busy, but all children need time to rest and recharge. If he suffers from any of the symptoms above, it might be time to cut back on what he's doing. Kids are often intensely motivated to make changes, particularly when they start their first part-time job, and he may go overboard. Keep an eye on his activity levels and make sure he has time to relax as well.

• Make sure that you have family time together, and that there is time for play and friends.

• Be physically affectionate with your child. The power of touch is well documented, and if your child feels loved and loveable, he'll feel good about himself and better able to withstand the effects of stress.

• Make sure your child isn't getting caffeine in his diet. Caffeine is found in chocolate and cola drinks, among other things, and it can increase adrenalin levels, enhancing the effects of stress.

• Encourage your child to think positively. Children are in training for facing the stresses of the adult world. Although all parents should make it their responsibility to keep their children's lives as stress-free as possible, it is important to teach life skills along the way. When things pile up, teach your child to plan ahead and to be optimistic, even when things go wrong.

• Ensure that your child gets plenty of exercise – and bear in mind that it should be fun!

• Encourage communication. The better your child is able to express his feelings and emotions, the more ably he will handle stress. If your child finds it hard to confide in you, see if you can find another family member or a teacher who can make some headway. Reassure him that it is OK to show how he feels – to cry or get angry. These are good ways of relieving tension and can make him feel better.

• Encourage your child to do things he enjoys, such as drawing, painting or writing, relaxing to music, or going to the cinema. Seeing friends, taking part in a sport or other leisure activity, and having their 'own space' to be alone are also important means of coping with stress.

Tantrums

Tantrums about food and eating are very common in many families, and most children are aware that food is an emotive issue. As a result, they use food as a weapon against their parents, and often have temper tantrums when they don't get what they want. So what drives a child to tantrum? In younger children, it is simply an inability to express the overpowering emotions they are feeling – they may be angry, hurt, frustrated, lonely or simply fed up. They do not have the skills to work out what it is they are feeling – they just act. Older children throw tantrums for attention, or because it embarrasses or distresses their parents to the point that they always give in.

How to cope

- The best way (which does take a lot of courage) is to ignore it completely. A child who gets no response by behaving in this type of uncontrolled way, will soon see that he needs to adopt a productive method of getting your attention. You are bound to get a lot of unwanted attention for ignoring a child, particularly in public places, but it is undoubtedly a technique that works. Some children have amazing tenacity and will continue long beyond the point where you thought she'd stop. But don't give in. Give in once, and you've planted that all important seed in her mind that she can use that technique again.

- Don't allow food to become an emotive issue and a reason for tantrums. If your child refuses to eat the food you serve, remove it and ignore any requests for a replacement. If she learns that tantrums over food aren't going to get her sweets and crisps instead of good healthy food, she'll eventually stop them.

- If it's too disruptive to allow a tantrum to continue (you may be at a restaurant, or in the supermarket), hug your child tightly, say that you love her, and then remove her from the scene. It might sound like rewarding problem behaviour by expressing love and affection, but your child may well feel out of control and need reassurance that everything is OK. The fact that her behaviour is not OK is something that you need to discuss later. For the time being, you need to deal with the tantrum itself.

- Don't be tempted to negotiate with a child in the throws of a tantrum. They are unlikely to listen to reason, and you'll probably end up becoming angry, which is counter-productive.

- Express understanding of the feeling they are experiencing, but make it clear that shows of temper are no way to deal with it. Ask them to think of better ways to show that they are angry, cross, tired or jealous.

- Be consistent. If you have a food policy in your house, you will need to stick to it. Don't give in to whining or tantrums, or you'll never get any peace. Stick to your guns and remain calm, but firm.

TV addicts

Kids who have spent a large proportion of their lives in front of the television may actually find that they need it. Lonely children in particular tend to view television programmes as 'friends' – and, indeed, they often take the place of them. Cutting your child's viewing habits dramatically may have an unexpectedly negative effect on your child – he may feel bereft, lonely, like he's missing out on something (the next instalment of his favourite soap or sitcom, for example) and very bored. He may even experience the equivalent of withdrawal symptoms, so don't be too harsh!

If your child loves TV, don't remove it from his life completely. Remember that TV is part of our popular culture, and denying him access to programmes that all of his friends are watching will make him feel left out. However, it is something that must be monitored carefully – just as you allow and discourage different types of foods. Every parent's job is to monitor such obsessions, without creating the forbidden-fruit syndrome where the child is so restricted, he craves the forbidden thing and sneaks around attempting to satisfy his insatiable desires.

Children are impulsive, they want what they want, when they want it. The parent's job is to help the child gain self-control and delay – and sometimes even deny – gratification of unhealthy physical and mental desires and demands.

TV, computers, games consoles and videos have an addictive effect – the more kids watch and play, the more they want to watch and play. So come up with some realistic and reasonable rules: one or two TV programmes each day; or an hour or two of anything 'media' in any given day. He'll have to make some choices. If there are more than a couple of hours of programmes he wants to watch, he can tape them and watch them another day. He's not then missing out, just delaying when he watches them. You can relax rules slightly on holidays and weekends, but ensure that there are still limits, or you'll never get your child off the sofa and out into the fresh air for some exercise.

Ultimately, as a parent you do need to make some choices for your children, on their behalf, and for health reasons. This is one of the most important ones you can make. He can choose his programming and scheduling within the rules you set down, but be firm. He'll eventually discover interests, and wonder why he was so obsessed in the first place (see also pages 159–161).

Resources

UK

Child health and fitness

Childline
Helpline: 0800 1111 (24 hours, for children only)
Website: www.childline.org.uk
Confidential help for children encountering problems at home or at school. Their website is an excellent source of information for parents, too, with plenty of advice on bullying and self-esteem issues that may be affecting your overweight child.

Discovery Health
Website: www.discoveryhealth.co.uk
A great resource for parents, with advice on all aspects of dealing with an overweight child.

Foodfitness
c/o Food and Drink Federation
6 Catherine Street
London WC2B 5JJ
Tel: 020 7836 2460
Fax: 020 7379 0481
Email: foodfitness@fdf.org.uk
Website: www.fdf.org.uk
Foodfitness is a healthy lifestyle initiative with a unique dual approach: promoting enjoyable, healthy eating combined with increased moderate physical activity. The aims of foodfitness are positive and non-judgemental and the five key messages are clear and understandable. The initiative is based on the philosophy that a healthy lifestyle is fun, easily achievable and affordable.

Healthy Living
Website: www.bbc.co.uk/health/healthyliving
A BBC site with lots of useful information about food and exercise for adults and children. Its 'Nutrition' section looks at the basics of healthy eating. Its 'Young People and Exercise' section has information about why it's good to be fit and ways of getting fit. It also addresses some of the excuses children make to avoid exercise. Visitors can work out their body mass index and use the Life Expectancy Calculator.

Institute of Child Health
University College London
30 Guilford Street
London WC1N 1EH
Tel: 020 7242 9789
Fax: 020 7831 0488
Website: www.ich.ucl.ac.uk
A wealth of information for parents and children on all types of health issues, with an excellent section on childhood obesity and overweight.

KidsHealth
Website: www.kidshealth.org
Excellent US site for children and teenagers about food and fitness. It includes a huge range of informative articles on everything from healthy snacks and what being the right weight means, to ways children can exercise on their own and how they can stay fit, even if they don't like sport.

Medical Research Council
20 Park Crescent
London W1B 1AL
Tel: 020 7636 5422
Fax: 020 7436 8112
Website: www.mrc.ac.uk
Information on research and issues involving overweight children, plus a look at policy changes required.

Move4Health
Website: www.move4health.org.uk
This UK organization campaigns to get more people, more active, more often.

Netdoctor
Website: www.netdoctor.co.uk
Plenty of good-quality information on all aspects of overweight, including advice on how to change eating habits and deal with associated problems.

Parents Jury
Tel: 020 7837 2250
Website: www.parentsjury.org.uk
The food industry claims only to sell products that parents want, but some parents are angry about the type of food sold for children and the way it is marketed. You can join them at the Parents Jury, an independent panel of parents which seeks to improve the quality of children's foods and drinks in the UK. The Jury is co-ordinated by The Food Commission, an independent watchdog that campaigns for healthier, safer food in the UK.

The Food Commission
Tel: 020 7837 2250
Website: www.foodcomm.org.uk
The Food Commission is a non-profit organization campaigning for the right to safe, wholesome food for all. It is largely funded by public subscriptions and donations and takes no subsidy from the government or food industry, allowing it to be completely independent. The Food Commission publishes *The Food Magazine*, full of tips and insights about food companies' techniques and tricks, and the latest consumer campaigns to hold them accountable.

TV Dinners: What's Being Served up by the Advertisers
Website: www.sustainweb.org/label1_childad.asp
This 2001 report from the food pressure group Sustain looks at the nature and extent of food advertising during children and adult viewing times. Among its findings was that children watching Saturday morning TV saw more than twice as many advertisements per hour for unhealthy foods as adults viewing after 9pm.

Counselling and emotional support

British Association for Behavioural and Cognitive Psychotherapies (BABCP)
The Globe Centre
PO Box 9
Accrington BB5 0XB
Tel: 01254 875 277
Website: www.babcp.com
Can provide details of accredited therapists.

British Association for Counselling and Psychotherapy (BACP)
BACP House
35–37 Albert Street
Rugby CV21 2SG
Tel: 0870 443 5252
Website: www.bacp.co.uk
See website or send A5 SAE for details of local practitioners.

Mind
Infoline: 0845 766 0163
Website: www.mind.org.uk
The leading mental health organization in England and Wales, Mind helps people with experience of mental distress to have a better quality of life. Plenty of good information for dealing with the emotional impact of overweight.

YoungMinds
102–108 Clerkenwell Road
London EC1M 5SA
Parents' information service: 0800 018 2138 (Any adult with concerns about the mental health of a child or young person can ring this service)
Website: www.youngminds.org.uk
Committed to improving the mental health of young people, this organization is an excellent source of information on the emotional aspects of growing up and dealing with overweight, and helps to deal with issues such as self-esteem, depression and bullying.

Eating disorders and overeating

Eating Disorders Association
103 Prince of Wales Road
Norwich NR1 1DW
Adult Helpline: 0845 634 1414 – Over 18 years of age
(open 8.30am–8.30pm Monday to Friday; 1.00pm–4.30pm Saturdays)
Youthline: 0845 634 7650 – Up to and including 18 years of age
(open 4.00pm–6.30pm Monday to Friday; 1.00pm–4.30pm Saturdays)
Email: hepmail@edauk.com (adults); talkback@edauk.com (youths)
Youthline e-mail service: talkback@edauk.com
Website: www.edauk.com
Information and help on all aspects of eating disorders including anorexia nervosa, bulimia nervosa, binge eating disorder and related eating disorders.

Overeaters Anonymous Great Britain
PO Box 19
Stretford
Manchester M32 9EB
Tel: 07000 784 985
Website: www.oagb.org.uk
Runs local groups throughout the country. Although aimed at adults at present, they can provide information and advice for parents of overweight children.

Educational resources

Breakfast Clubs
Website: www.breakfast-club.co.uk
Encourages schools to set up clubs that offer children a balanced meal at the start of each school day. It aims to get pupils thinking about the value of a more nutritional diet as they experience the benefits of healthy food. The site has downloadable resources to support developing a club. These include information on funding, and case studies.

Coolmeals
Website: www.coolmeals.co.uk
Information on health and nutrition particularly aimed at seven to 11-year-olds. Among its features is the interactive 'Virtual Body Lab', where children can see how their diet, the amount of exercise they do and their general lifestyle affects them physically and mentally. Visuals also allow them to see what happens in their body when nutrients such as calcium are consumed. Advice is then given on how they can improve their diet and lifestyle.

Dish It Up!
Tel: 0845 606 0667
Email: foodstandards@eclogistics.co.uk
This free, fun-filled CD-Rom from the Food Standards Agency is aimed at 11 to 12-year-olds and is packed with information and interactive games and quizzes. It has been developed to foster positive attitudes towards healthy eating and lifestyle by experiencing a 'virtual' day in the life of a young person. To order contact Food Standards Agency Publications.

Football Association
Website: www.thefa.com/grassroots/footballinschools
The FA website has resources and programmes to develop skills at all levels. Its primary school section has information about TOP Sport, which aims to develop football in the PE curriculum for seven to 11-year-olds. There's also a cross-curricular resource pack for key stage 2 that's based on the FA Cup.

Grab 5!
Website: www.grab5.com
Grab 5! is a project which provides help and ideas for primary schools wanting to encourage their pupils to eat more fruit and vegetables. The project is co-ordinated by the food pressure group Sustain.

Join the Activaters
Tel: 020 7836 2460
Website: www.foodfitness.org.uk
This free, interactive CD-Rom for seven to nine-year-olds is from the Food and Drink Federation. It aims to promote the basic principles of enjoyable healthy eating and exercise through the cartoon families the Activaters and the Dolittles.

Media Smart
Website: www.mediasmart.org.uk/kids
Teaches children aged six to 11 about how television advertising works. It helps them develop the skills to interpret, understand and think critically about the ads they see. A downloadable resource that's particularly suitable for the literacy hour features a teaching video, poster, teachers' notes, activity sheets and leaflet for parents.

Nutrition Explorations

Website: www.nutritionexplorations.org

This US site has useful news and information about the latest research into nutrition. It also features a section for parents, as well as educational games for children.

The Food Dudes

Website: www.fooddudes.co.uk

The Food Dudes programme, developed by psychologists at the University of Wales Bangor, is a successful initiative for use in primary schools to encourage and maintain healthy eating habits. Children enjoy the Food Dudes and both teachers and parents have praised the positive, long-term effect the programme has on children's diet.

Walk to School

Website: www.walktoschool.org.uk

The National Walk to School initiative aims to get children to participate in this activity. It features teaching ideas for literacy, numeracy and local studies, and its 'Walkabout' download has a further 100 or so cross-curricular ideas, and photocopiable activity sheets. There are also sections for pupils where they can read fun facts and about other children's walking experiences.

Wired For Health

Website: www.wiredforhealth.gov.uk

Has information and resources linked to the national curriculum and the National Healthy School Standards. It also features four fun health sites for young people aged five to 16, which include games, quizzes and information.

Nutrition

The British Dietetic Association

5th Floor Charles House

148/9 Great Charles Street

Queensway

Birmingham B3 3HT

Tel: 0121 200 8080

Fax: 0121 200 8081

E-mail: info@bda.uk.com

Website: www.bda.uk.com

Formed to provide training and facilities for dietitians, the Association can give you advice on finding a dietitian or other nutrition expert, as well as general advice on dealing with obesity in children.

The British Nutrition Foundation
High Holborn House
52–54 High Holborn
London WC1V 6RQ
Tel: 020 7404 6504
Fax: 020 7404 6747
Email: postbox@nutrition.org.uk
Website: www.nutrition.org.uk
An extremely helpful source of information and advice for parents, covering all aspects
of food and diet, as well as regular news updates.

Food Standards Agency
Aviation House
125 Kingsway
London WC2B 6NH
Switchboard: 020 7276 8000
Website: www.foodstandards.gov.uk
Plenty of good information on all aspects of food and health, including an invalu-
able section on food allergies and sensitivities. Lots of up-to-date research, informa-
tion about health concerns, diets, food labelling and more. Worth a visit.

The Institute for Optimum Nutrition
13 Blades Court
Deodar Road
London SW15 2NU
Tel: 020 8877 9993
Website: www.ion.ac.uk
Good nutrition through education and personal consultation.

Obesity

Association for the Study of Obesity (ASO)
Website: www.aso.org.uk
The ASO promotes research into the causes, prevention and treatment of obesity, encourages action to reduce obesity, and can put you into contact with organizations interested in obesity and weight regulation. An excellent source of good-quality information
and advice for parents of overweight children.

International Association for the Study of Obesity
incorporating the International Obesity Task Force (IOTF)
231 North Gower Street
London NW1 2NS
Tel: 020 7691 1900
Fax: 020 7387 6033
E-mail: inquiries@iaso.org and/or obesity@iotf.org
Website: www.iaso.org and/or www.iotf.org
The IOTF is working to alert the world of the growing health crisis threatened by soaring levels of obesity. You'll find news, research, information and excellent links.

National Obesity Forum
PO Box 6625
Nottingham NG2 5PA
Tel/Fax: 0115 8462109
Website: www.nationalobesityforum.org.uk
The National Obesity Forum was established in May 2000 to raise awareness of the growing impact of obesity and overweight. Although it is an organization of healthcare professionals, it provides an invaluable source of information for the general public as well, and offers good links and research.

Weight Concern
Brook House
2–16 Torrington Place
London
WC1E 7HN
Tel: 020 7679 6636
Fax: 020 7813 2848
E-mail: enquiries@weightconcern.com
Website: www.weightconcern.com
A registered charity, this organization helps to address the physical and psychological needs of overweight and obese people of all ages. They have an excellent website, with research, facts and stats, weight calculators, dietary information and more. They also provide a reliable source of information on issues relating to obesity, including prejudice and misinformation.

Specific health issues

Allergy UK
Deepdene House
30 Bellegrove Road
Welling
Kent DA16 3PY
Website: www.allergyfoundation.com
A good source of information plus links to organizations who can help with food sensitivities.

ASH (Action on Smoking and Health)
102–108 Clifton Street
London EC2A 4HW
Tel: 020 7739 5902
Website: www.ash.org.uk
An excellent source of information and advice on giving up smoking and helping young people to do so, too. Lots of facts, stats and good links.

British Heart Foundation
14 Fitzhardinge Street
London W1H 6DH
Tel: 020 7935 0185
Heart Information Line: 08450 70 80 70
Website: www.bhf.org.uk
Good source of information on heart disease related to obesity and overweight, including dietary and exercise advice.

Cancer Research UK
PO Box 123
Lincoln's Inn Fields
London WC2A 3PX
Tel (Customer Services): 020 7009 8820
Fax: 020 7269 3100
Website: www.cancerresearch.org.uk
Good information on cancers related to diet and overweight, plus dietary advice, research, links and overall help.

Diabetes UK
10 Parkway
London NW1 7AA
Tel: 020 7424 1000
Diabetes UK Careline: 0845 120 2960, 9–5, Monday to Friday
Fax: 020 7424 1001
Email: info@diabetes.org.uk
Website: www.diabetes.org.uk
Information and advice on all aspects of dealing with diabetes.

Sleep Matters
Medical Advisory Service
PO Box 3087
London W4 4ZP
Helpline: 020 8994 9874
Help for children with sleep problems.

The British Snoring and Sleep Apnoea Association
'The Steps'
How Lane
Chipstead
Surrey CR5 3LT
Provides information for sufferers and their families. Please send a large sae.

Other resources

Australia

ABC's Active Kids Australia
Website: www.activekidz.com.au
Includes fun pages, recipes and advice on fitness.

ASH Australia
PO Box 572
Kings Cross 1340
Tel: 02 9334 1876
Fax: 02 9334 1742
Email: annej@ashaust.org.au
Website: www.ashaust.org.au
Information on the dangers of smoking and advice on helping teenagers give up.

Better Health Channel
Website: www.betterhealth.vic.gov.au
Information, advice and lots of articles on obesity and overweight.

DepressioNet
Website: www.depressionet.com.au
Good information and support for those with depression and their families.

Diabetes Australia
Level 5
39 London Circuit
Canberra City ACT 2600
Helpline: 1300 136 588
Fax: 61 2 6230 1535
Email: cccp@diabetesaustralia.com.au
Website: www.diabetesaustralia.com.au
Information and advice on all aspects of diabetes.

Eating Disorders Foundation of Victoria
1513 High Street
Glen Iris
Victoria 3146
Tel: 03 9885 0318
Fax: 03 9885 1153
Email: edfv@eatingdisorders.org.au
Website: www.eatingdisorders.org.au
Support and information for those with eating disorders and their carers.

Fresh for Kids
Website: www.freshforkids.com.au
Great interactive food website for kids.

International Association for the Study of Obesity
incorporating the International Obesity Task Force (IOTF)
Asia-Pacific Office
Human Nutrition Unit
University of Sydney NSW 2006
Tel: 61 2 9351 3758
Website: www.iotf.org
News, research and information on obesity.

Nutrition Australia
Australian Capital Territory
PO Box 5146
Garran ACT 2605
Email: act@NutritionAustralia.org
Website: www.nutritionaustralia.org
Community-based organization providing advice on nutrition with the aim of encouraging healthy eating.

New Zealand

Agencies for Nutrition Action
Tel: 03 374 6909
Fax: 03 379 6125
Email: ana@cph.co.nz
Website: www.ana.org.nz
Group aiming to tackle obesity through the promotion of good nutrition and physical activity.

Diabetes New Zealand
PO Box 12 441
Thorndon
Wellington
Tel: 04 499 7145
Fax: 04 499 7146
Email: admin@diabetes.org.nz
Website: www.diabetes.org.nz
Information for those with diabetes and those at risk.

Eating Disorders Services
PO Box 13 807
Johnsonville
Wellington
Tel: 04 478 6674
Fax: 04 477 4160
Email: info@eatingdisorders.org.nz
Website: www.eatingdisorders.org.nz
Services for people with eating disorders, their families, and schools.

New Zealand Dietetic Association
PO Box 5065
Wellington
Tel: 04 473 3061
Email: nzda@dietitians.org.nz
Website: www.dietitians.org.nz
Help with finding a dietitian, nutritional information and plenty of links.

National Heart Foundation
Website: www.nhf.org.nz
Useful information for parents, kids and schools on healthy eating and exercise.

Sport and Recreation New Zealand
Website: www.sparc.org.nz
Encourages sport and an active life, and includes a section for kids.

Singapore

Trim and Fit (TAF)
Website: www.moe.gov.sg (go to curriculum/programmes)
A Ministry of Education programme started in 1992 to help tackle childhood obesity.

South Africa

Cancer Association of South Africa
www.cansa.org.za

Glycemic Index Foundation of South Africa (GIFSA)
www.gifoundation.com

Health Care Directory
www.medpages.co.za

Heart Foundation of South Africa
www.heartfoundation.co.za

International Diabetes Federation
www.idf.org

Mental Health Information Centre of South Africa (includes eating disorders)
www.sun.ac.za/mentalhealth

Index

OTHER RODALE BOOKS
AVAILABLE FROM PAN MACMILLAN

1-4050-4182-X	The Doctors' Book of Home Remedies	*A Prevention Health Book*	£20.00
1-4050-0675-7	The Secret Life of the Dyslexic Child	*Robert Frank Ph.D with Kathryn E. Livingston*	£10.99
1-4050-6721-7	Balancing Pregnancy and Work	*Nancy Hall with Karen Sullivan*	£12.99
1-4050-2097-0	Six Questions That Can Change Your Life	*Joseph Nowinski*	£8.99
1-4050-4191-9	Healing the Hurt Restoring the Hope	*Suzy Marta*	£12.99
1-4050-3340-1	When Your Body Gets the Blues	*Marie-Annette Brown & Jo Robinson*	£10.99

All Pan Macmillan titles can be ordered from our website, *www.panmacmillan.com*, or from your local bookshop and are also available by post from:

Bookpost, PO Box 29, Douglas, Isle of Man IM99 1BQ
Tel: 01624 836000; fax: 01624 670923; e-mail: *bookshop@enterprise.net*;
or visit: *www.bookpost.co.uk*. Credit cards accepted. Free postage and packing in the United Kingdom

Prices shown above were correct at time of going to press.
Pan Macmillan reserve the right to show new retail prices on covers which may differ from those previously advertised in the text or elsewhere.

For information about buying *Rodale* titles in **Australia**, contact Pan Macmillan Australia.
Tel: 1300 135 113; fax: 1300 135 103; e-mail: *customer.service@macmillan.com.au*;
or visit: *www.panmacmillan.com.au*

For information about buying *Rodale* titles in **New Zealand**, contact Macmillan Publishers
New Zealand Limited. Tel: (09) 414 0356; fax: (09) 414 0352;
e-mail: *lyn@macmillan.co.nz*;
or visit: *www.macmillan.co.nz*

For information about buying *Rodale* titles in **South Africa**, contact Pan Macmillan
South Africa. Tel: (011) 325 5220; fax: (011) 325 5225;
e-mail: *roshni@panmacmillan.co.za*